Face Charts
for
Makeup Artists

PLAN. PRACTICE. RECORD.

wandering tortoise

ISBN: 978-1679635212

Design/Client Name ____________ Date ____________

Concealer	Brows
Foundation	Lid Color 1
Contour	Lid Color 2
Blush	Lid Color 3
Highlights	Crease
Powder	Lip Liner
Eye Liner	Lip Color
Mascara	Lip Gloss

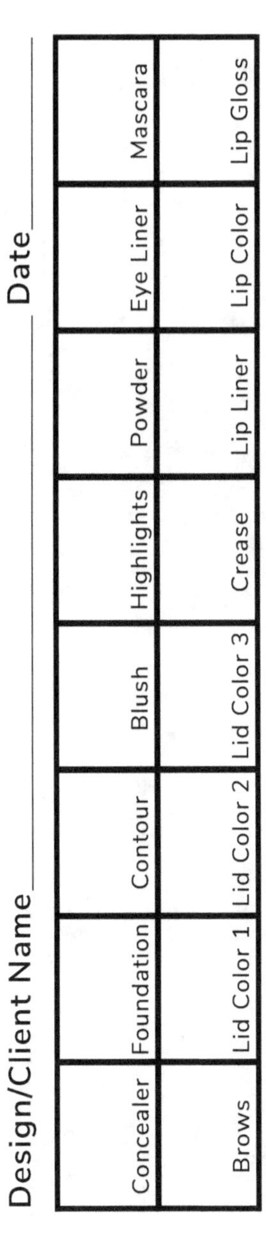

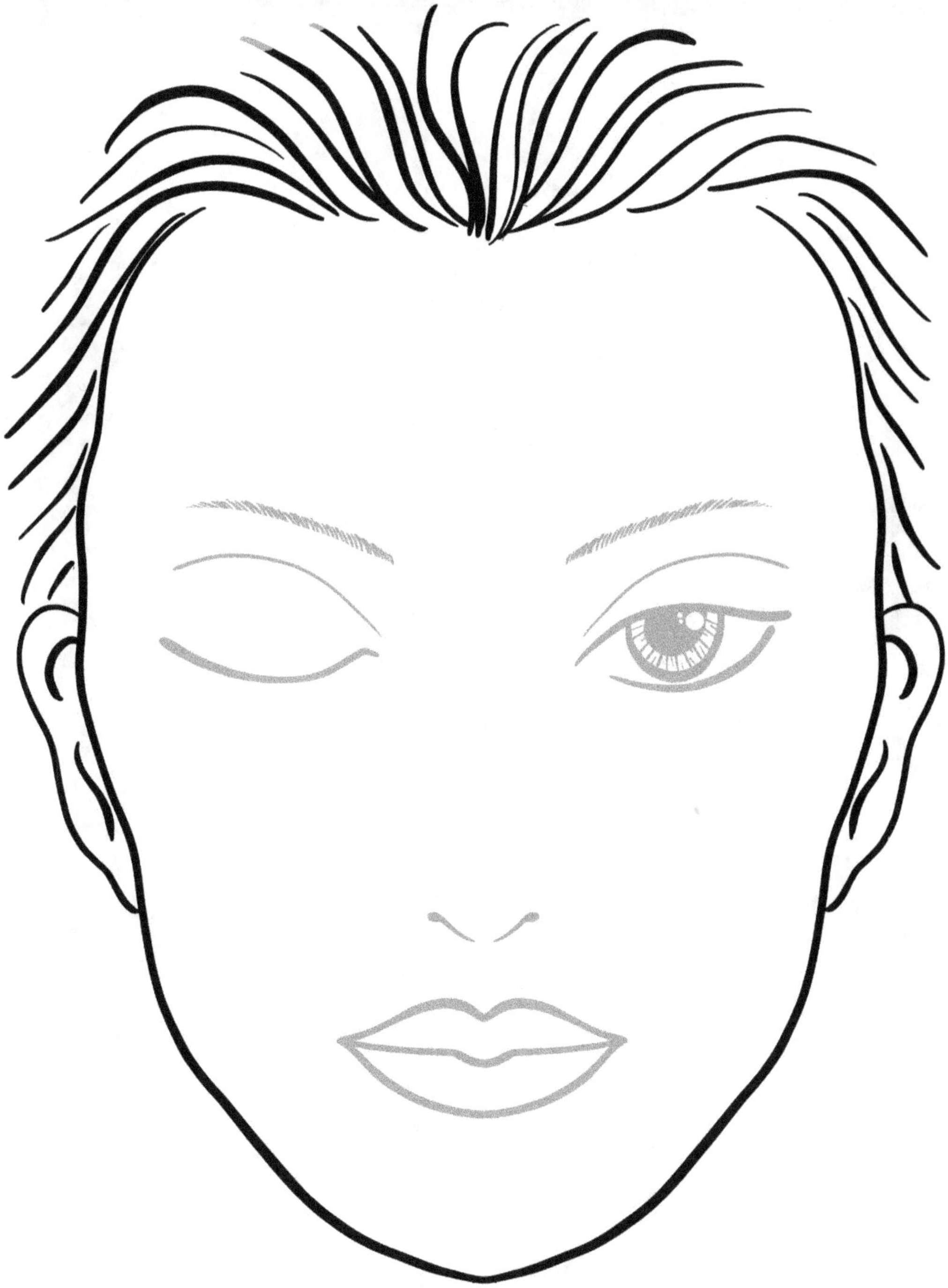

Details

Skin Tone ____________________

Eye Color ____________________

Hair Color ____________________

Lips (color, brand, etc.)

Lip Liner ____________________

Lip Color ____________________

Gloss ____________________

Eyes (color, brand, etc.)

Brows ____________________

Lid Color 1 ____________________

Lid Color 2 ____________________

Lid Color 3 ____________________

Crease ____________________

Eye Liner ____________________

Mascara ____________________

Face (color, brand, etc.)

Concealer ____________________

Foundation ____________________

Contour ____________________

Blush ____________________

Highlights ____________________

Powder ____________________

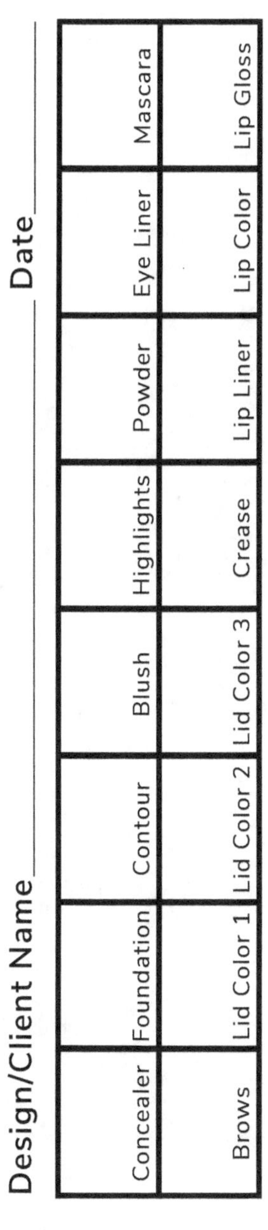

Date _______

Design/Client Name _______

Mascara	Lip Gloss
Eye Liner	Lip Color
Powder	Lip Liner
Highlights	Crease
Blush	Lid Color 3
Contour	Lid Color 2
Foundation	Lid Color 1
Concealer	Brows

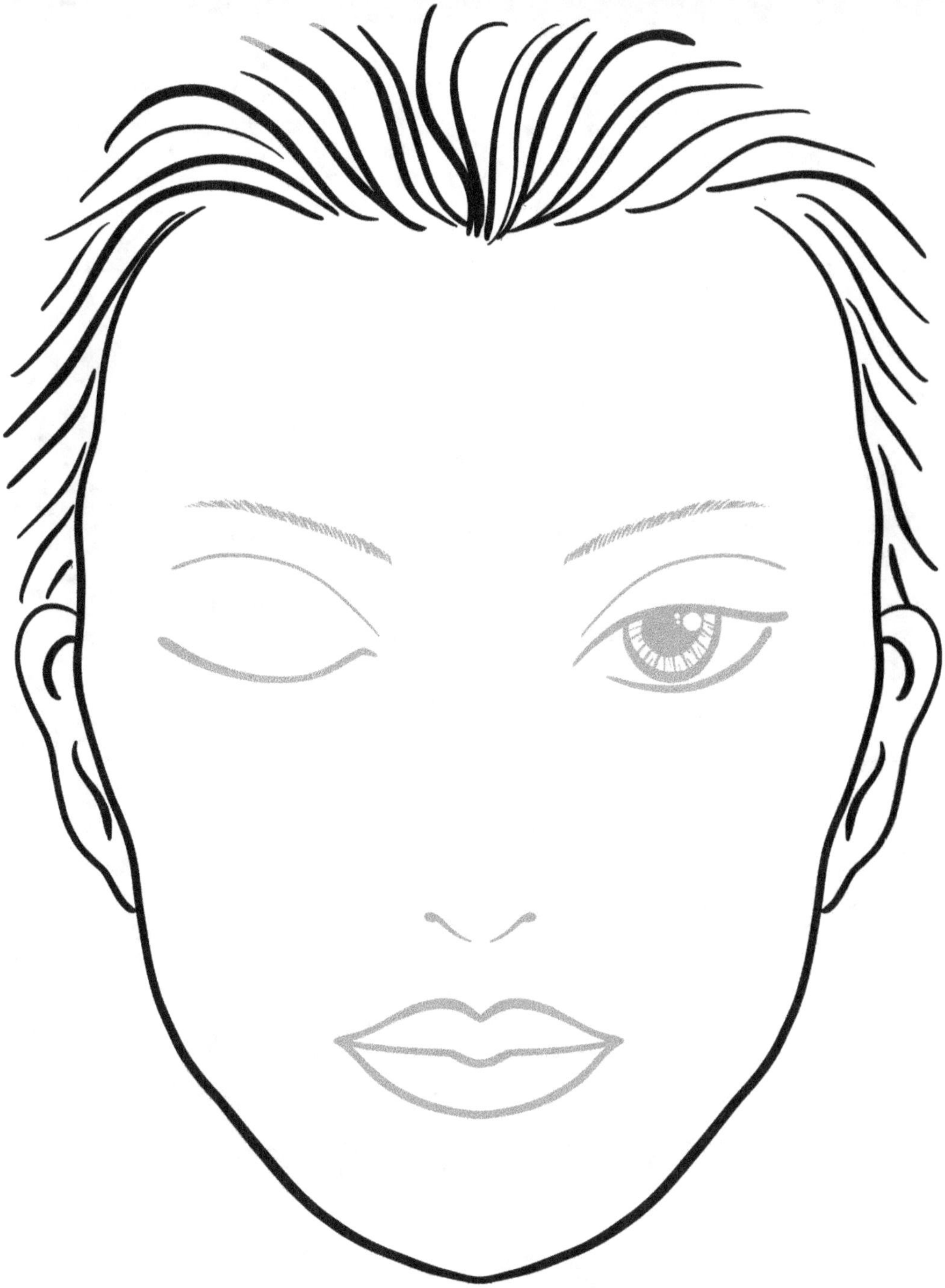

Details

Skin Tone _______________________

Eye Color _______________________

Hair Color _______________________

Lips (color, brand, etc.)

Lip Liner _______________________

Lip Color _______________________

Gloss _______________________

Eyes (color, brand, etc.)

Brows _______________________

Lid Color 1 _______________________

Lid Color 2 _______________________

Lid Color 3 _______________________

Crease _______________________

Eye Liner _______________________

Mascara _______________________

Face (color, brand, etc.)

Concealer _______________________

Foundation _______________________

Contour _______________________

Blush _______________________

Highlights _______________________

Powder _______________________

Date _______________

Design/Client Name _______________

Mascara	Lip Gloss
Eye Liner	Lip Color
Powder	Lip Liner
Highlights	Crease
Blush	Lid Color 3
Contour	Lid Color 2
Foundation	Lid Color 1
Concealer	Brows

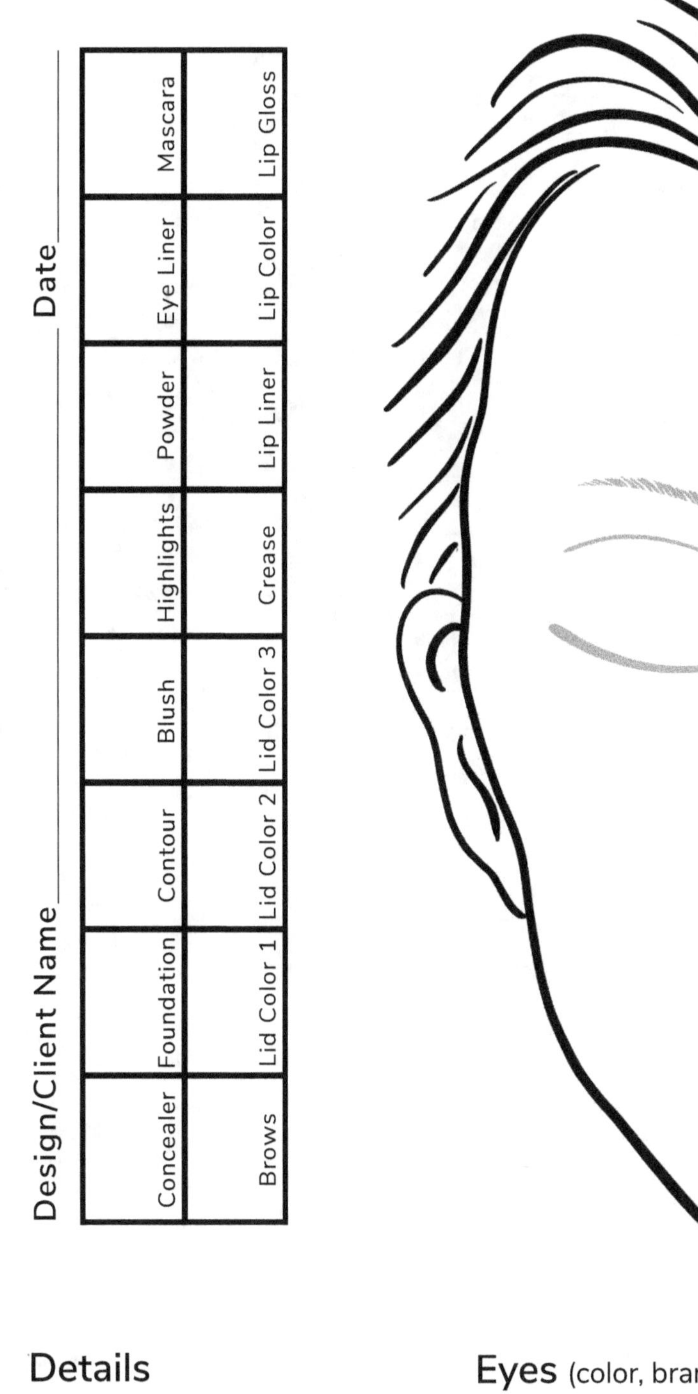

Details

Skin Tone _______________

Eye Color _______________

Hair Color _______________

Lips (color, brand, etc.)

Lip Liner _______________

Lip Color _______________

Gloss _______________

Eyes (color, brand, etc.)

Brows _______________

Lid Color 1 _______________

Lid Color 2 _______________

Lid Color 3 _______________

Crease _______________

Eye Liner _______________

Mascara _______________

Face (color, brand, etc.)

Concealer _______________

Foundation _______________

Contour _______________

Blush _______________

Highlights _______________

Powder _______________

Design/Client Name______________________ Date______

Concealer	Foundation	Contour	Blush	Highlights	Powder	Eye Liner	Mascara
Brows	Lid Color 1	Lid Color 2	Lid Color 3	Crease	Lip Liner	Lip Color	Lip Gloss

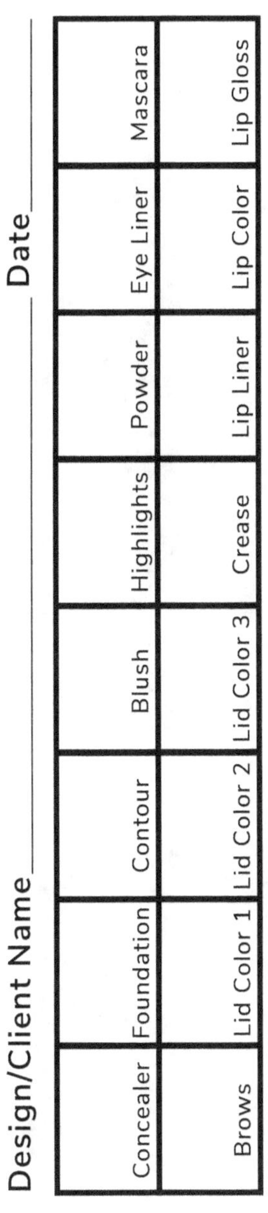

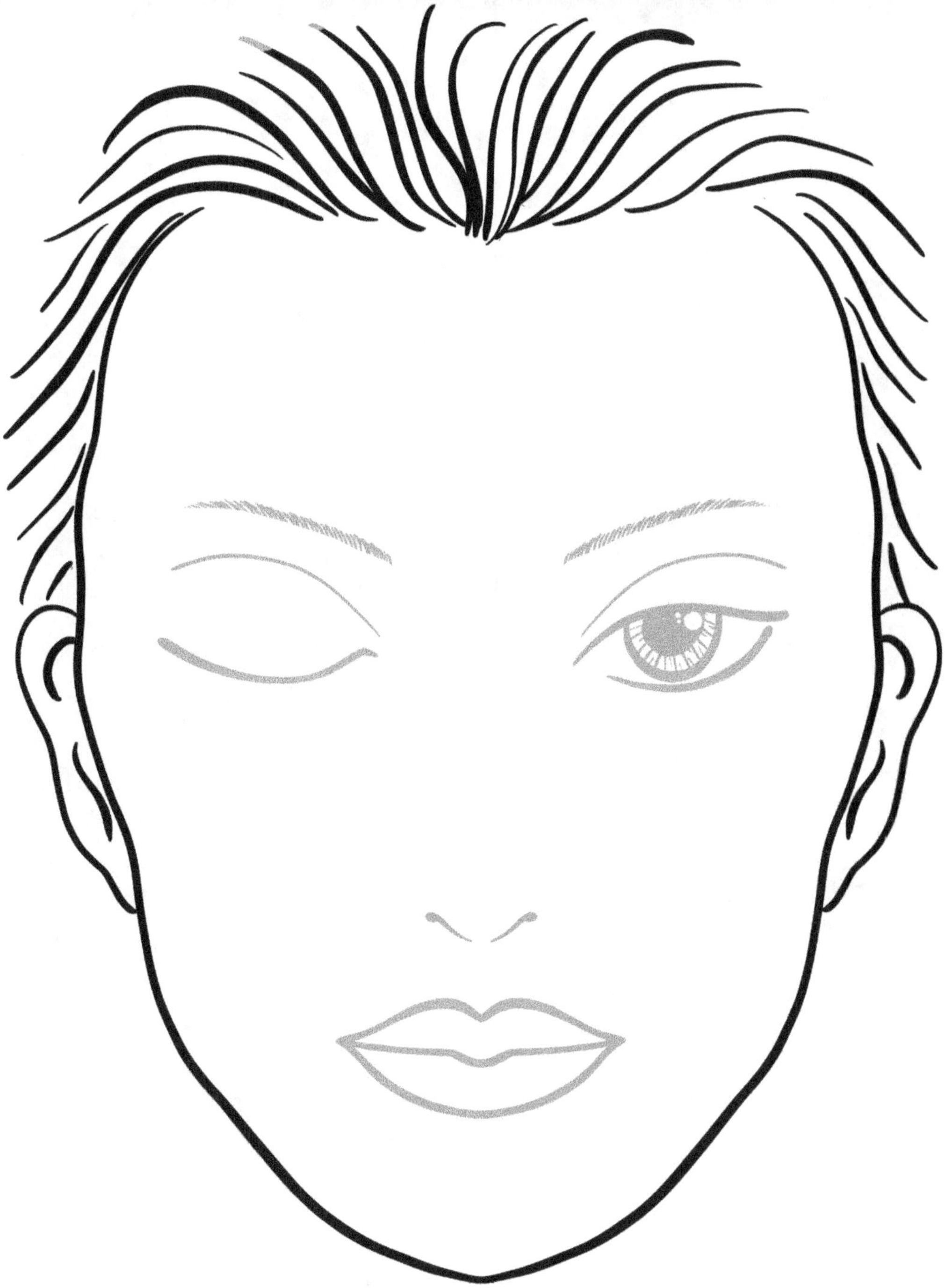

Details

Skin Tone____________________

Eye Color ____________________

Hair Color____________________

Lips (color, brand, etc.)

Lip Liner ____________________

Lip Color ____________________

Gloss ____________________

Eyes (color, brand, etc.)

Brows ____________________

Lid Color 1 ____________________

Lid Color 2 ____________________

Lid Color 3 ____________________

Crease____________________

Eye Liner____________________

Mascara ____________________

Face (color, brand, etc.)

Concealer____________________

Foundation____________________

Contour____________________

Blush ____________________

Highlights ____________________

Powder____________________

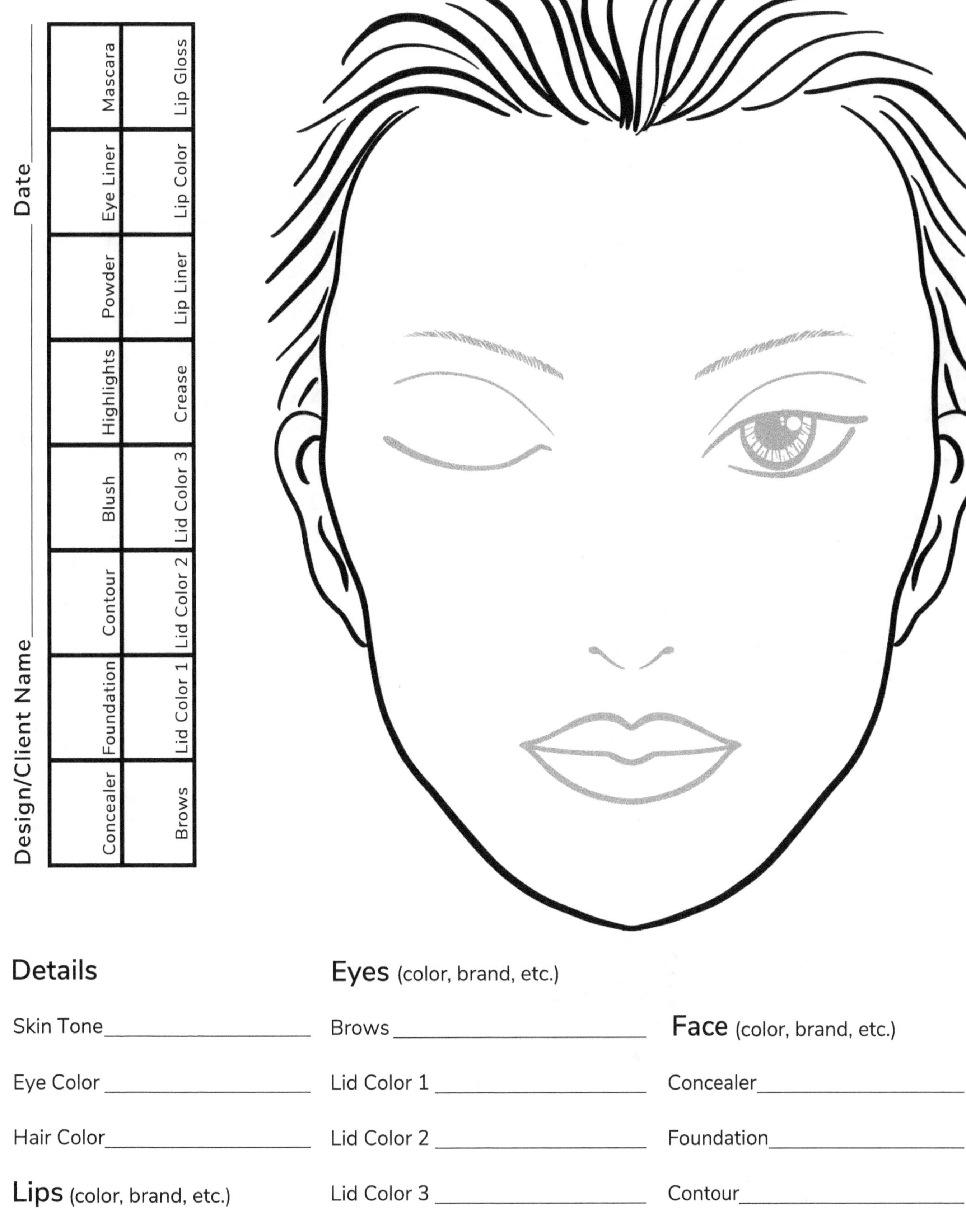

Details

Skin Tone _______________________

Eye Color _______________________

Hair Color _______________________

Lips (color, brand, etc.)

Lip Liner _______________________

Lip Color _______________________

Gloss _______________________

Eyes (color, brand, etc.)

Brows _______________________

Lid Color 1 _______________________

Lid Color 2 _______________________

Lid Color 3 _______________________

Crease _______________________

Eye Liner _______________________

Mascara _______________________

Face (color, brand, etc.)

Concealer _______________________

Foundation _______________________

Contour _______________________

Blush _______________________

Highlights _______________________

Powder _______________________

Design/Client Name_______________ Date__________

Concealer	Foundation	Contour	Blush	Highlights	Powder	Eye Liner	Mascara
Brows	Lid Color 1	Lid Color 2	Lid Color 3	Crease	Lip Liner	Lip Color	Lip Gloss

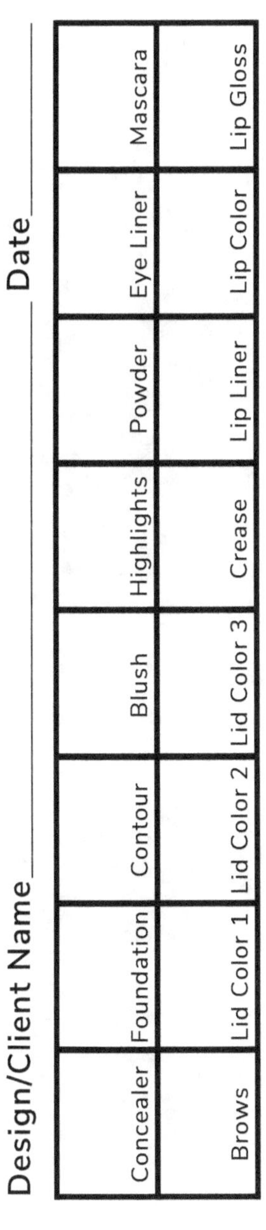

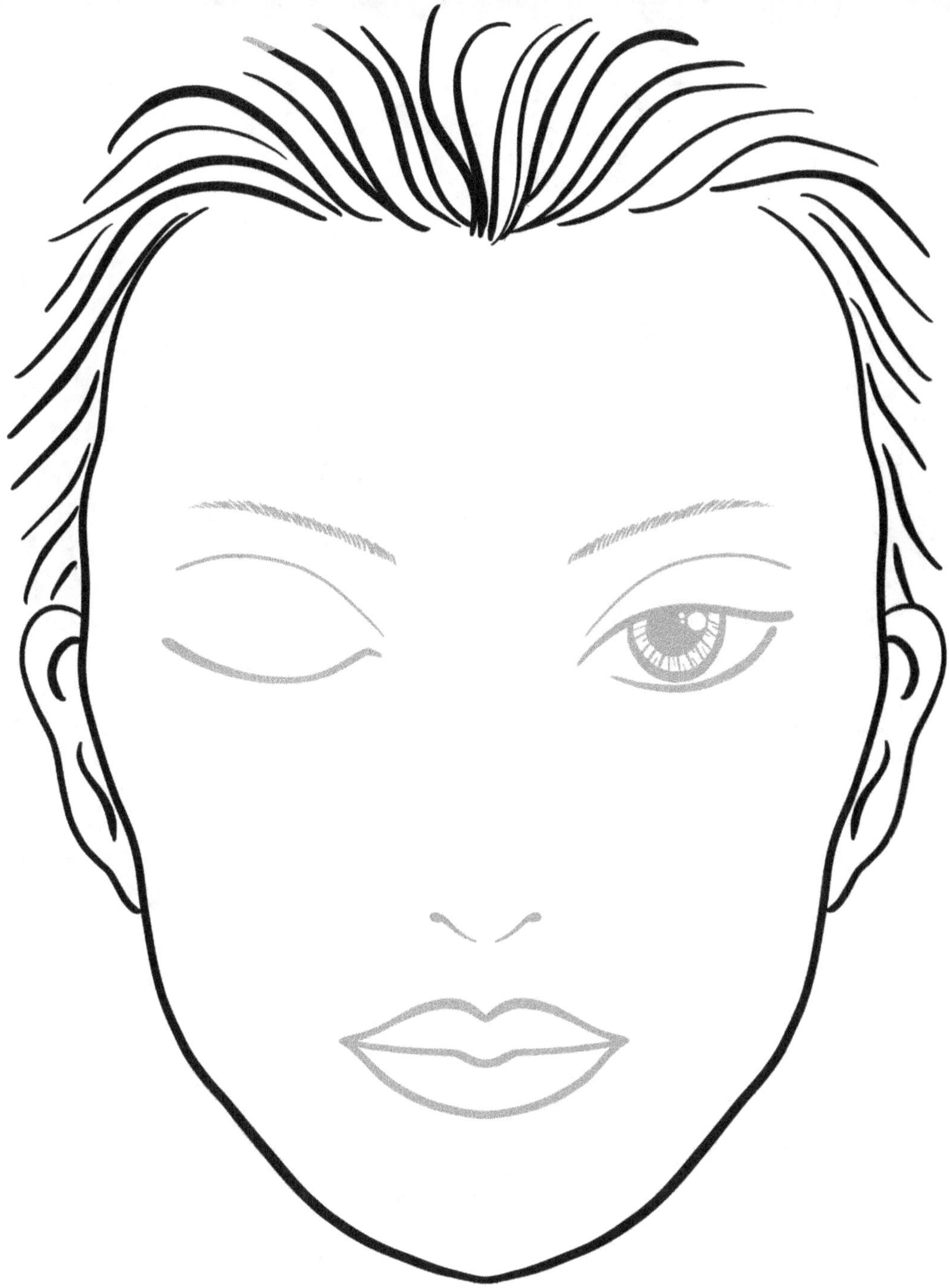

Details

Skin Tone____________________

Eye Color ____________________

Hair Color____________________

Lips (color, brand, etc.)

Lip Liner ____________________

Lip Color ____________________

Gloss ____________________

Eyes (color, brand, etc.)

Brows ____________________

Lid Color 1 ____________________

Lid Color 2 ____________________

Lid Color 3 ____________________

Crease ____________________

Eye Liner____________________

Mascara ____________________

Face (color, brand, etc.)

Concealer____________________

Foundation____________________

Contour____________________

Blush ____________________

Highlights ____________________

Powder____________________

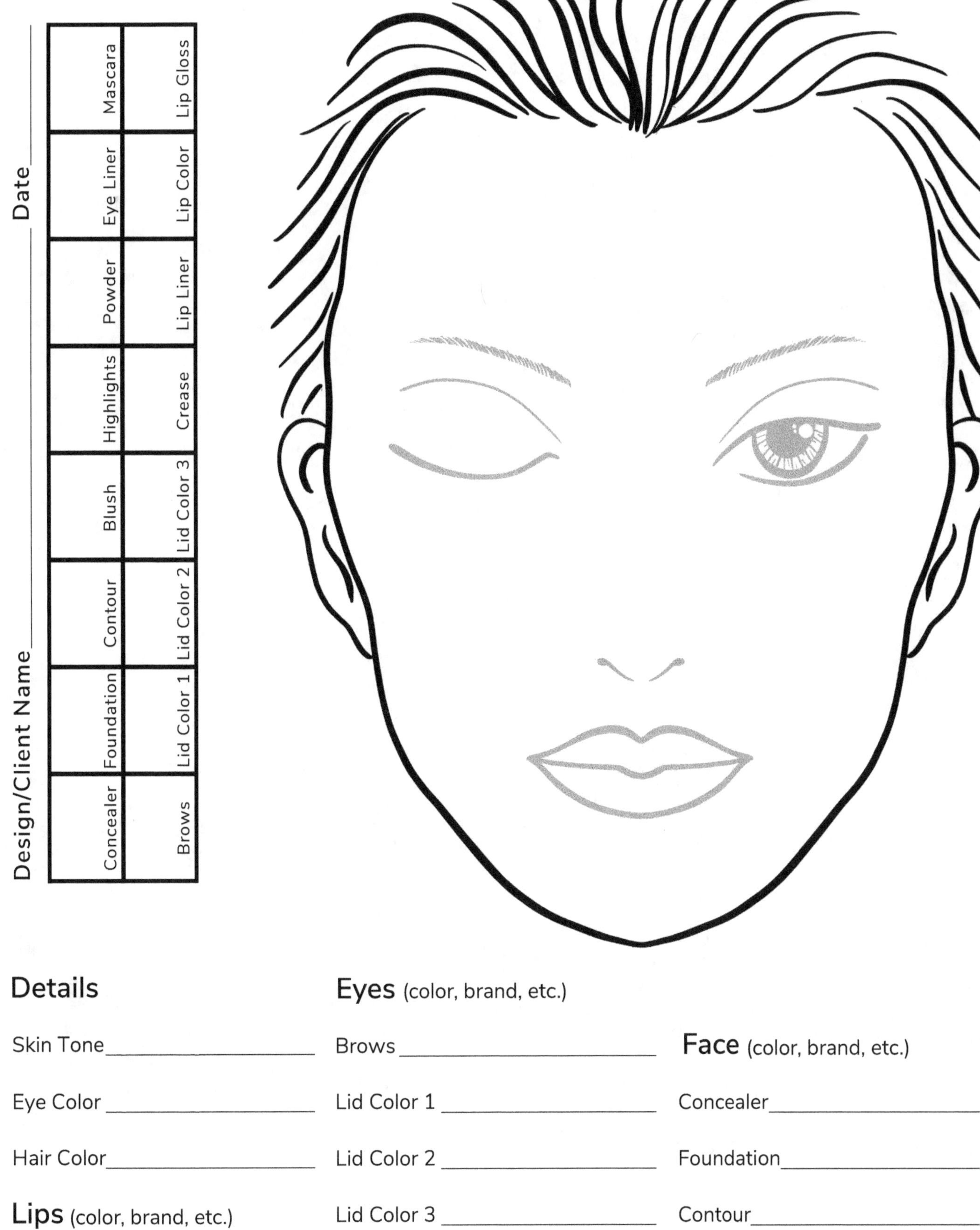

Details

Skin Tone _______________________

Eye Color _______________________

Hair Color _______________________

Lips (color, brand, etc.)

Lip Liner _______________________

Lip Color _______________________

Gloss _______________________

Eyes (color, brand, etc.)

Brows _______________________

Lid Color 1 _______________________

Lid Color 2 _______________________

Lid Color 3 _______________________

Crease _______________________

Eye Liner _______________________

Mascara _______________________

Face (color, brand, etc.)

Concealer _______________________

Foundation _______________________

Contour _______________________

Blush _______________________

Highlights _______________________

Powder _______________________

Design/Client Name_______________ Date_______________

Concealer	Foundation	Contour	Blush	Highlights	Powder	Eye Liner	Mascara
Brows	Lid Color 1	Lid Color 2	Lid Color 3	Crease	Lip Liner	Lip Color	Lip Gloss

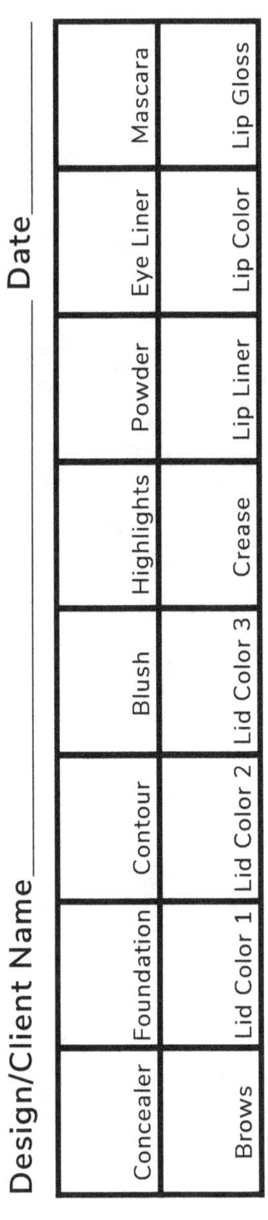

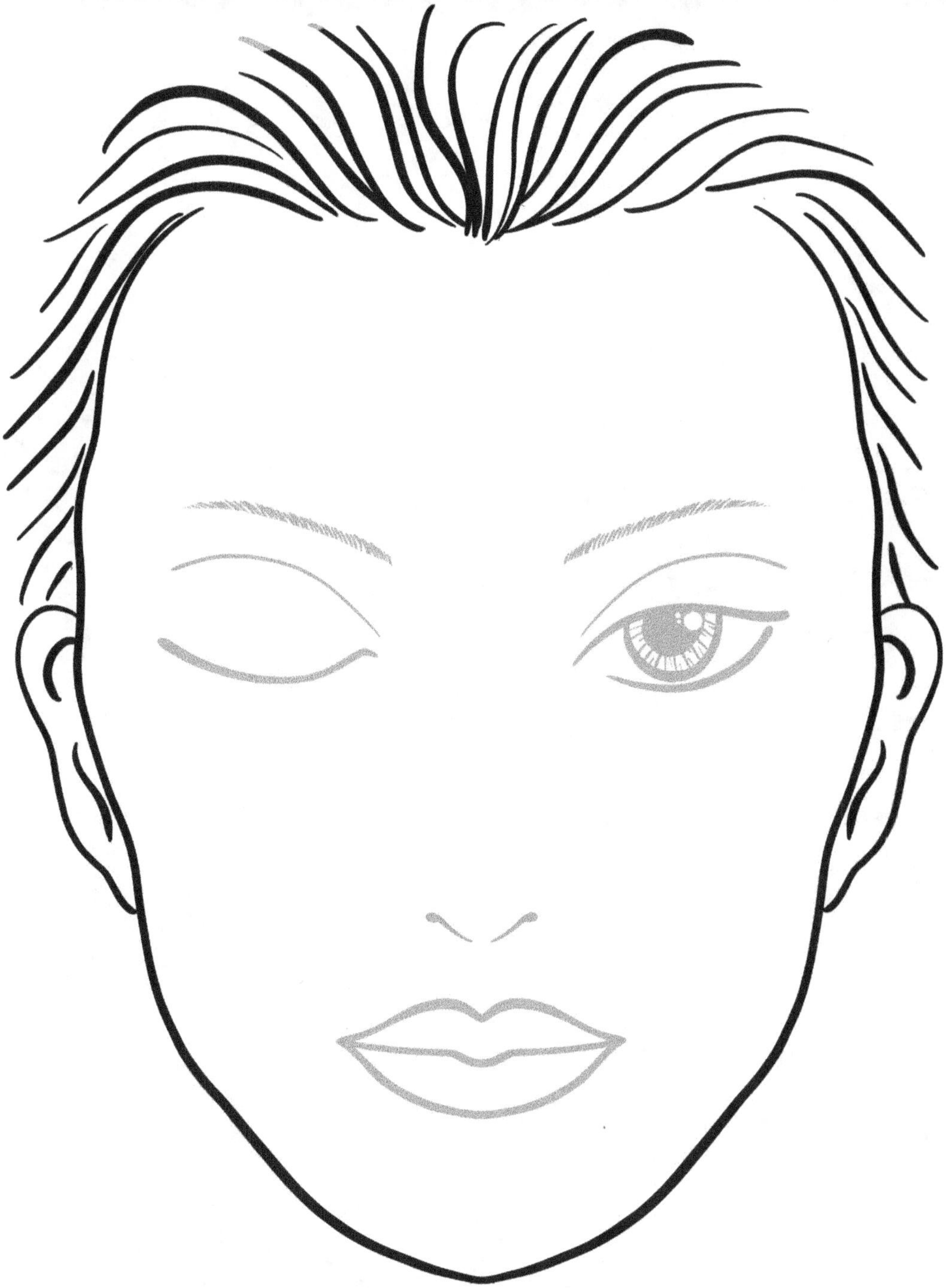

Details

Skin Tone_______________

Eye Color _______________

Hair Color_______________

Lips (color, brand, etc.)

Lip Liner _______________

Lip Color _______________

Gloss _______________

Eyes (color, brand, etc.)

Brows _______________

Lid Color 1 _______________

Lid Color 2 _______________

Lid Color 3 _______________

Crease _______________

Eye Liner_______________

Mascara _______________

Face (color, brand, etc.)

Concealer_______________

Foundation_______________

Contour_______________

Blush _______________

Highlights _______________

Powder_______________

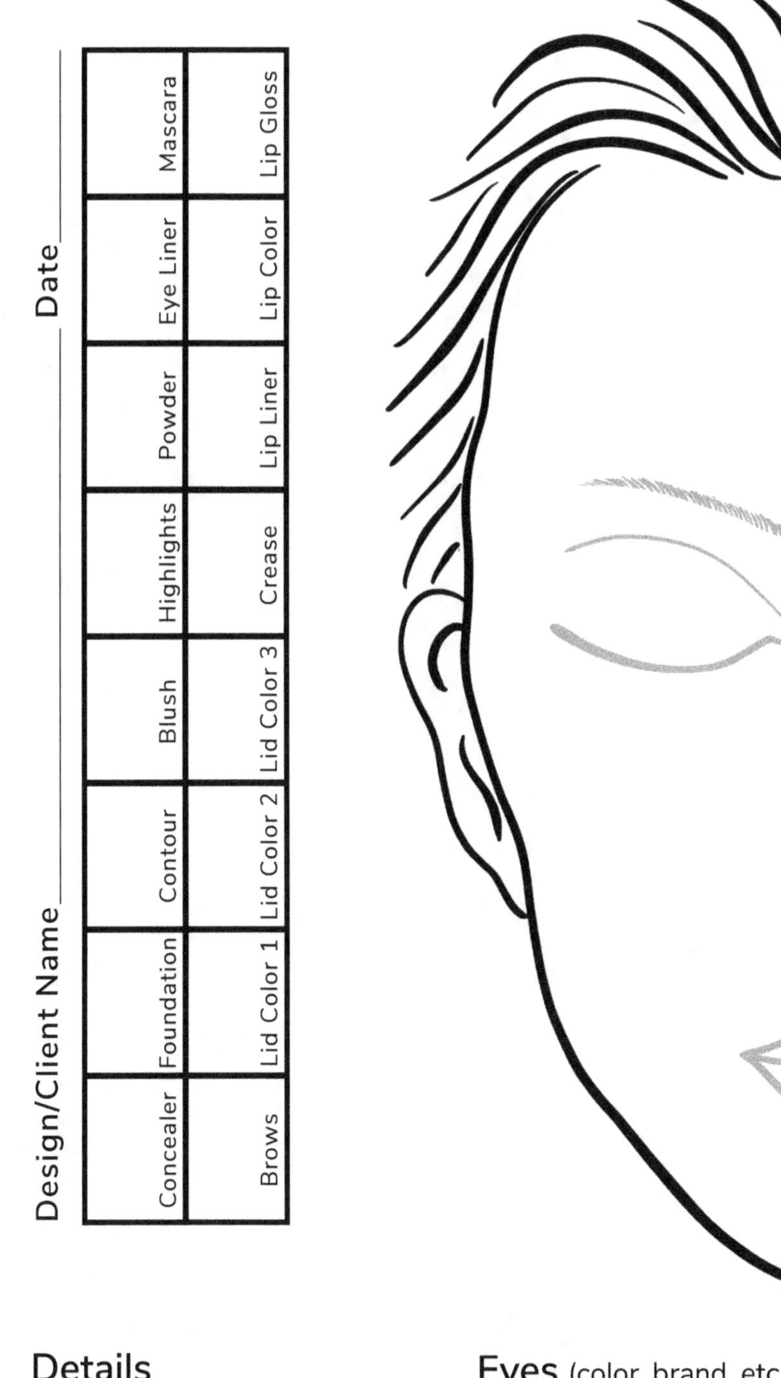

Details

Skin Tone ___________________

Eye Color ___________________

Hair Color ___________________

Lips (color, brand, etc.)

Lip Liner ___________________

Lip Color ___________________

Gloss ___________________

Eyes (color, brand, etc.)

Brows ___________________

Lid Color 1 ___________________

Lid Color 2 ___________________

Lid Color 3 ___________________

Crease ___________________

Eye Liner ___________________

Mascara ___________________

Face (color, brand, etc.)

Concealer ___________________

Foundation ___________________

Contour ___________________

Blush ___________________

Highlights ___________________

Powder ___________________

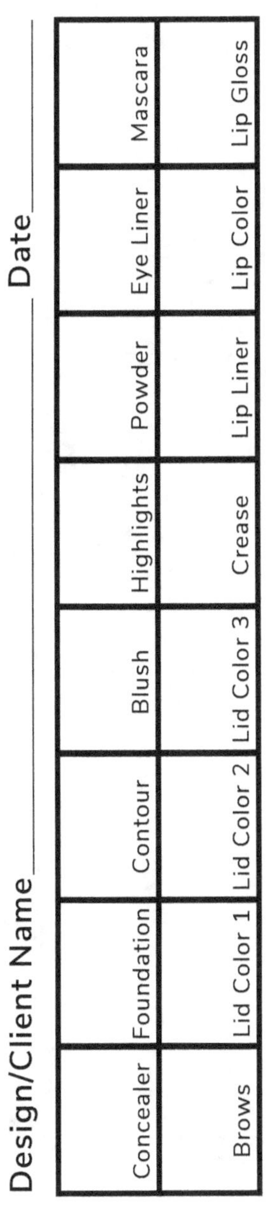

Date __________

Design/Client Name __________

Concealer	Foundation	Contour	Blush	Highlights	Powder	Eye Liner	Mascara
Brows	Lid Color 1	Lid Color 2	Lid Color 3	Crease	Lip Liner	Lip Color	Lip Gloss

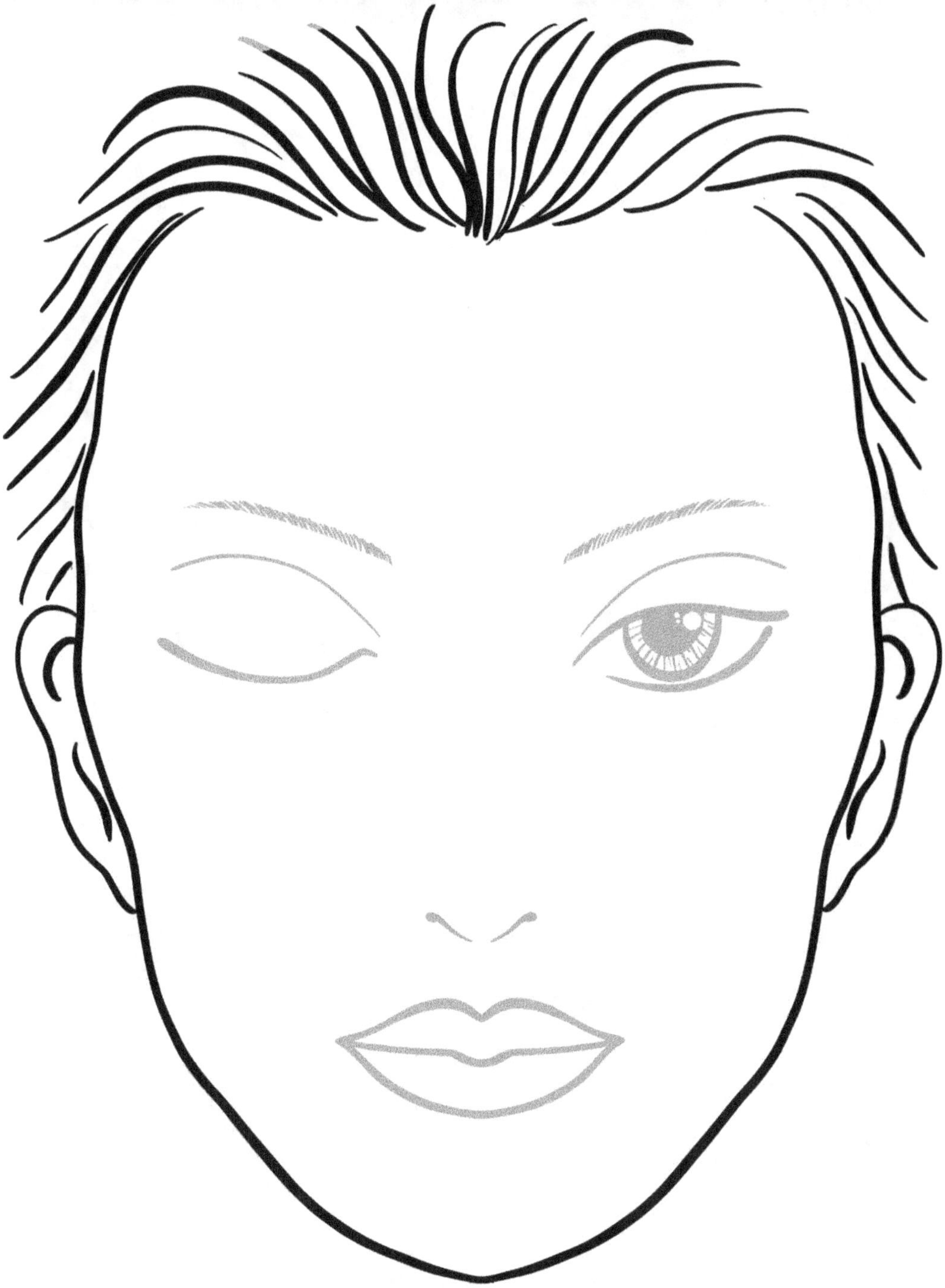

Details

Skin Tone __________________

Eye Color __________________

Hair Color __________________

Lips (color, brand, etc.)

Lip Liner __________________

Lip Color __________________

Gloss __________________

Eyes (color, brand, etc.)

Brows __________________

Lid Color 1 __________________

Lid Color 2 __________________

Lid Color 3 __________________

Crease __________________

Eye Liner __________________

Mascara __________________

Face (color, brand, etc.)

Concealer __________________

Foundation __________________

Contour __________________

Blush __________________

Highlights __________________

Powder __________________

Design/Client Name____________ Date____________

Concealer	Foundation	Contour	Blush	Highlights	Powder	Eye Liner	Mascara
Brows	Lid Color 1	Lid Color 2	Lid Color 3	Crease	Lip Liner	Lip Color	Lip Gloss

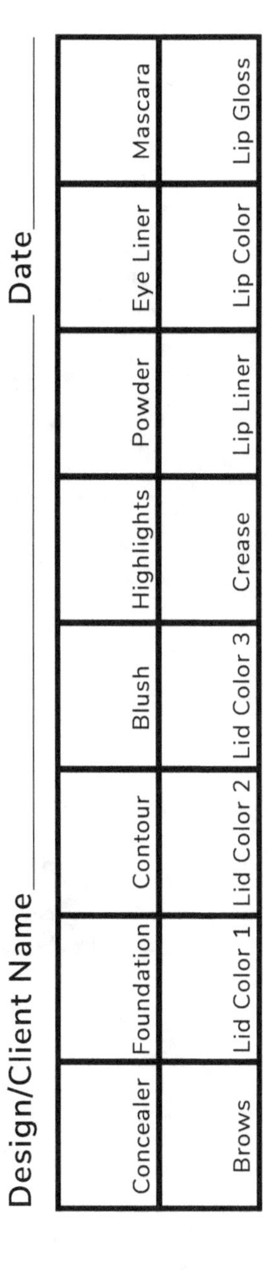

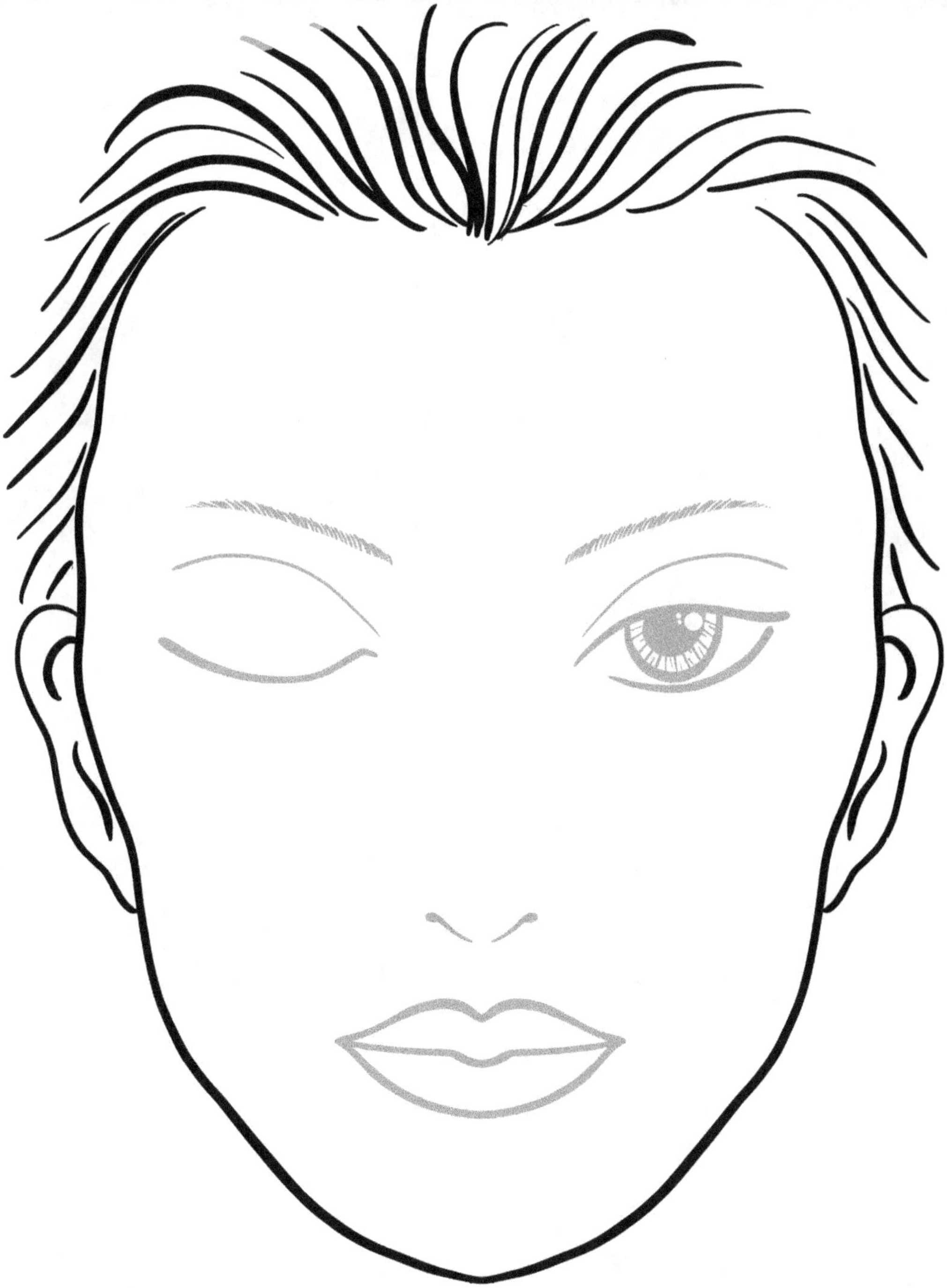

Details

Skin Tone____________________

Eye Color ____________________

Hair Color____________________

Lips (color, brand, etc.)

Lip Liner ____________________

Lip Color ____________________

Gloss ____________________

Eyes (color, brand, etc.)

Brows ____________________

Lid Color 1 ____________________

Lid Color 2 ____________________

Lid Color 3 ____________________

Crease____________________

Eye Liner____________________

Mascara ____________________

Face (color, brand, etc.)

Concealer____________________

Foundation____________________

Contour____________________

Blush ____________________

Highlights ____________________

Powder____________________

Design/Client Name ____________ Date ____________

Concealer	Foundation	Contour	Blush	Highlights	Powder	Eye Liner	Mascara
Brows	Lid Color 1	Lid Color 2	Lid Color 3	Crease	Lip Liner	Lip Color	Lip Gloss

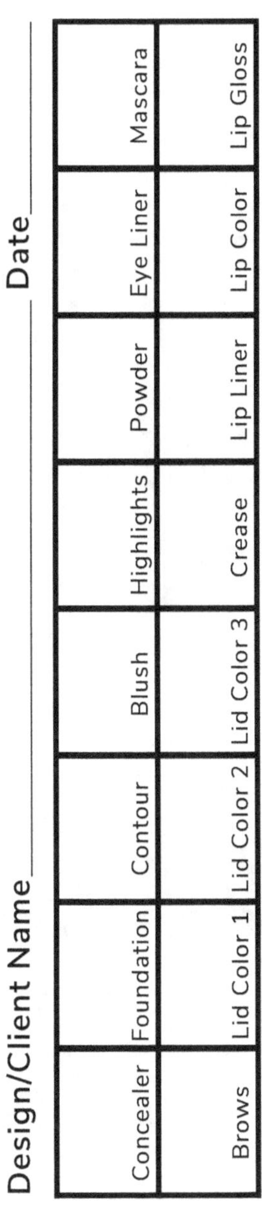

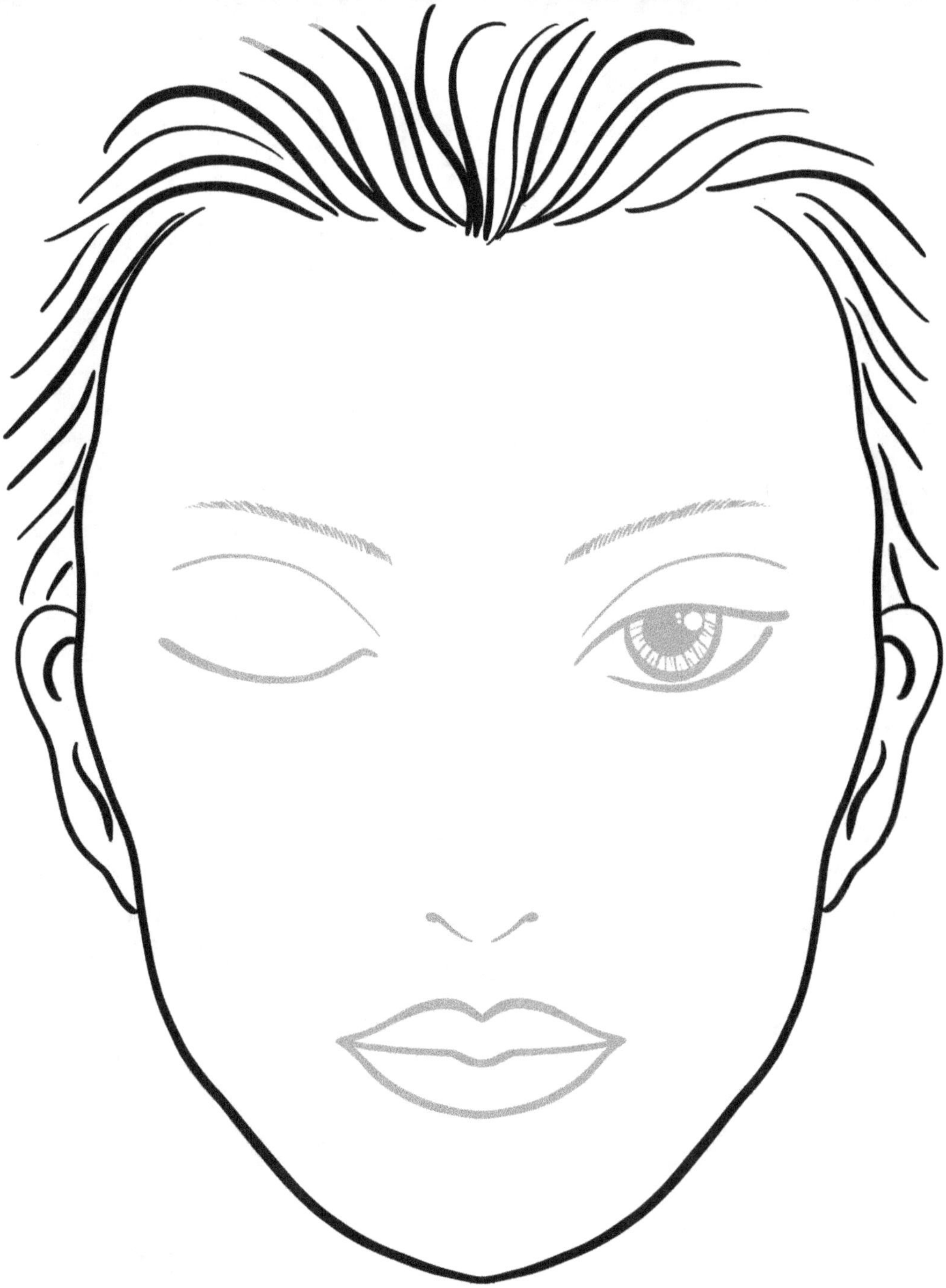

Details

Skin Tone ____________________

Eye Color ____________________

Hair Color ____________________

Lips (color, brand, etc.)

Lip Liner ____________________

Lip Color ____________________

Gloss ____________________

Eyes (color, brand, etc.)

Brows ____________________

Lid Color 1 ____________________

Lid Color 2 ____________________

Lid Color 3 ____________________

Crease ____________________

Eye Liner ____________________

Mascara ____________________

Face (color, brand, etc.)

Concealer ____________________

Foundation ____________________

Contour ____________________

Blush ____________________

Highlights ____________________

Powder ____________________

Design/Client Name________ Date________

Concealer	Foundation	Contour	Blush	Highlights	Powder	Eye Liner	Mascara
Brows	Lid Color 1	Lid Color 2	Lid Color 3	Crease	Lip Liner	Lip Color	Lip Gloss

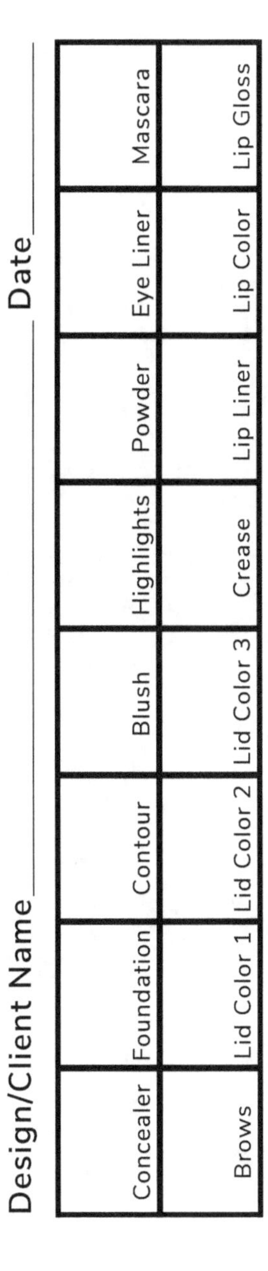

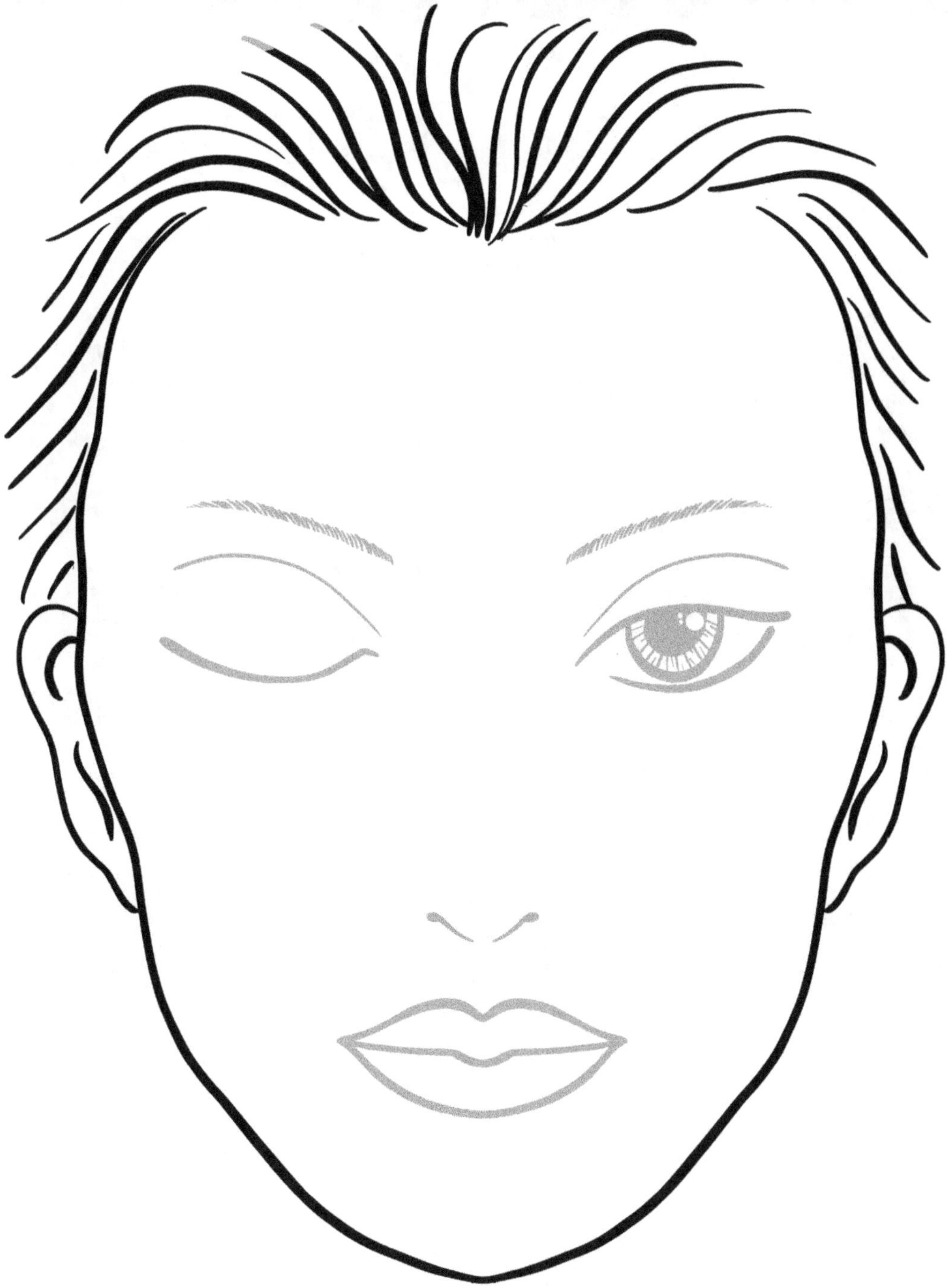

Details

Skin Tone____________________

Eye Color ____________________

Hair Color____________________

Lips (color, brand, etc.)

Lip Liner ____________________

Lip Color ____________________

Gloss ____________________

Eyes (color, brand, etc.)

Brows ____________________

Lid Color 1 ____________________

Lid Color 2 ____________________

Lid Color 3 ____________________

Crease____________________

Eye Liner____________________

Mascara ____________________

Face (color, brand, etc.)

Concealer____________________

Foundation____________________

Contour____________________

Blush ____________________

Highlights ____________________

Powder____________________

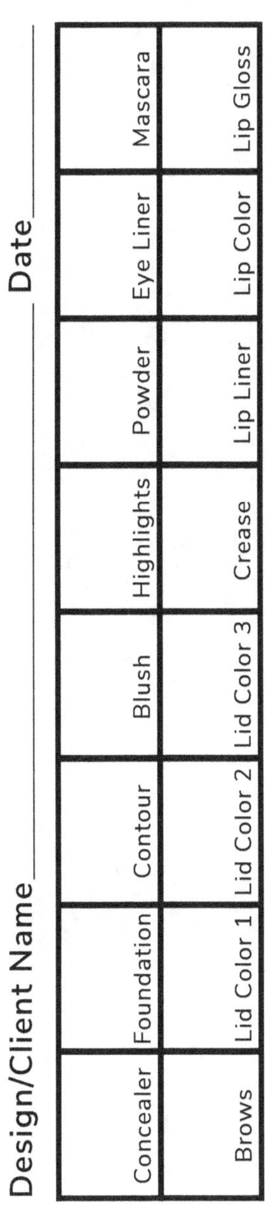

Date ___

Design/Client Name ___

Concealer	Foundation	Contour	Blush	Highlights	Powder	Eye Liner	Mascara
Brows	Lid Color 1	Lid Color 2	Lid Color 3	Crease	Lip Liner	Lip Color	Lip Gloss

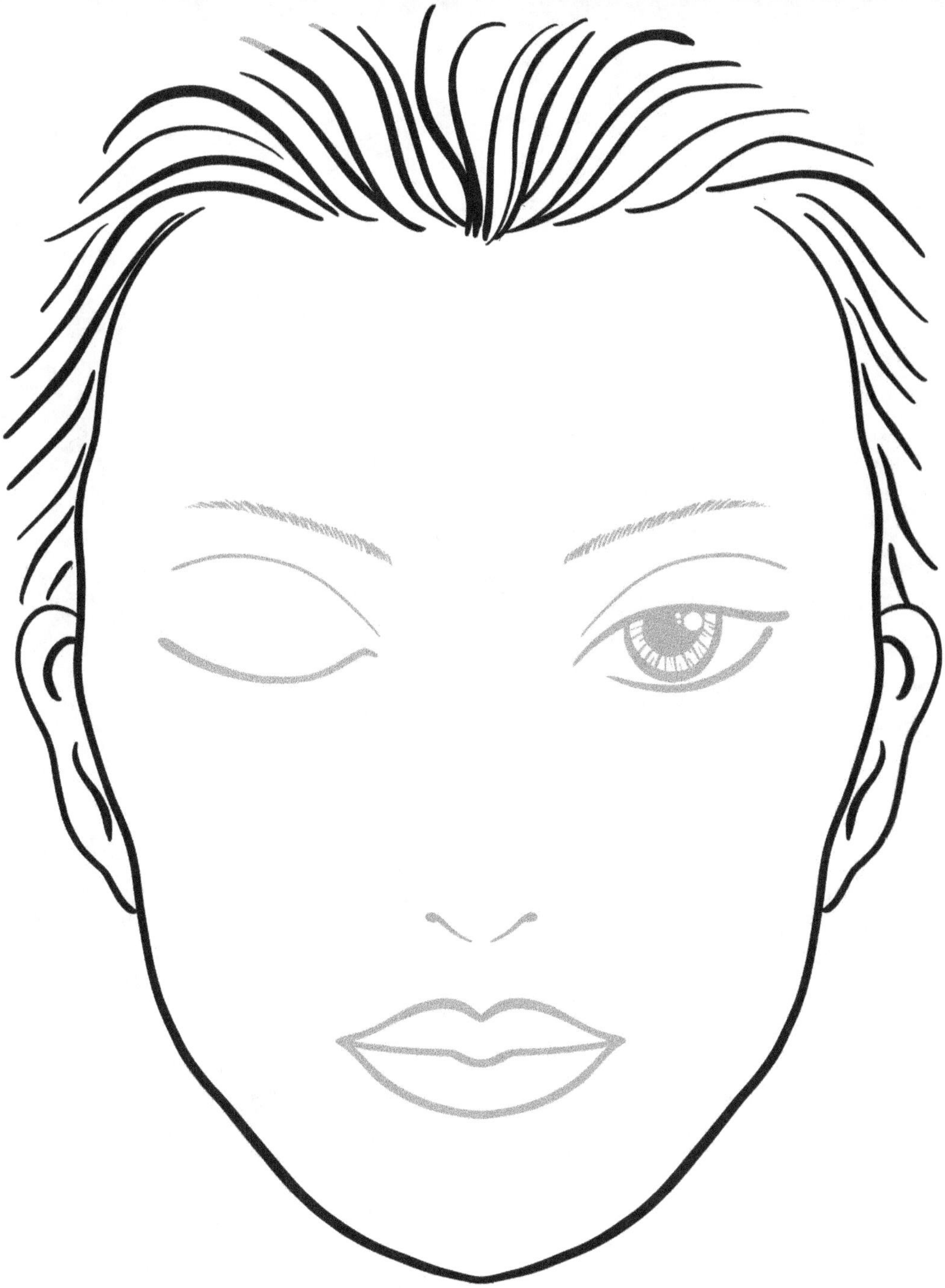

Details

Skin Tone _______________________

Eye Color _______________________

Hair Color _______________________

Lips (color, brand, etc.)

Lip Liner _______________________

Lip Color _______________________

Gloss _______________________

Eyes (color, brand, etc.)

Brows _______________________

Lid Color 1 _______________________

Lid Color 2 _______________________

Lid Color 3 _______________________

Crease _______________________

Eye Liner _______________________

Mascara _______________________

Face (color, brand, etc.)

Concealer _______________________

Foundation _______________________

Contour _______________________

Blush _______________________

Highlights _______________________

Powder _______________________

Concealer	Foundation	Contour	Blush	Highlights	Powder	Eye Liner	Mascara
	Lid Color 1	Lid Color 2	Lid Color 3	Crease	Lip Liner	Lip Color	Lip Gloss
Brows							

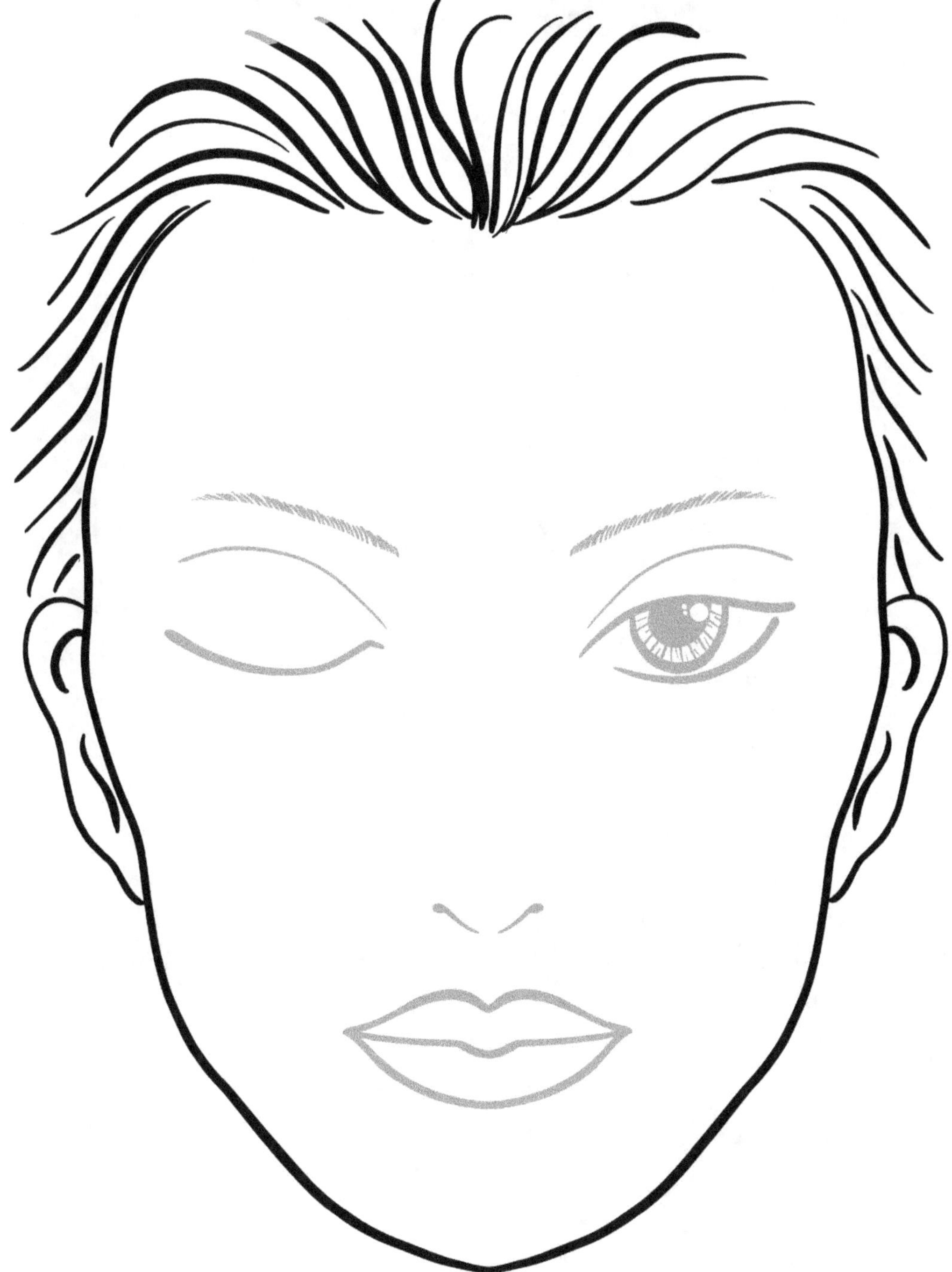

Details

Skin Tone _____________________

Eye Color _____________________

Hair Color _____________________

Lips (color, brand, etc.)

Lip Liner _____________________

Lip Color _____________________

Gloss _____________________

Eyes (color, brand, etc.)

Brows _____________________

Lid Color 1 _____________________

Lid Color 2 _____________________

Lid Color 3 _____________________

Crease _____________________

Eye Liner _____________________

Mascara _____________________

Face (color, brand, etc.)

Concealer _____________________

Foundation _____________________

Contour _____________________

Blush _____________________

Highlights _____________________

Powder _____________________

Design/Client Name ____________________ Date ____________

Concealer	Foundation	Contour	Blush	Highlights	Powder	Eye Liner	Mascara
Brows	Lid Color 1	Lid Color 2	Lid Color 3	Crease	Lip Liner	Lip Color	Lip Gloss

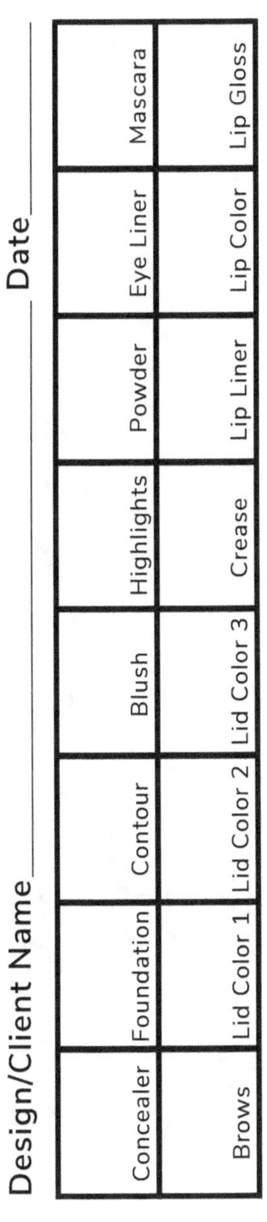

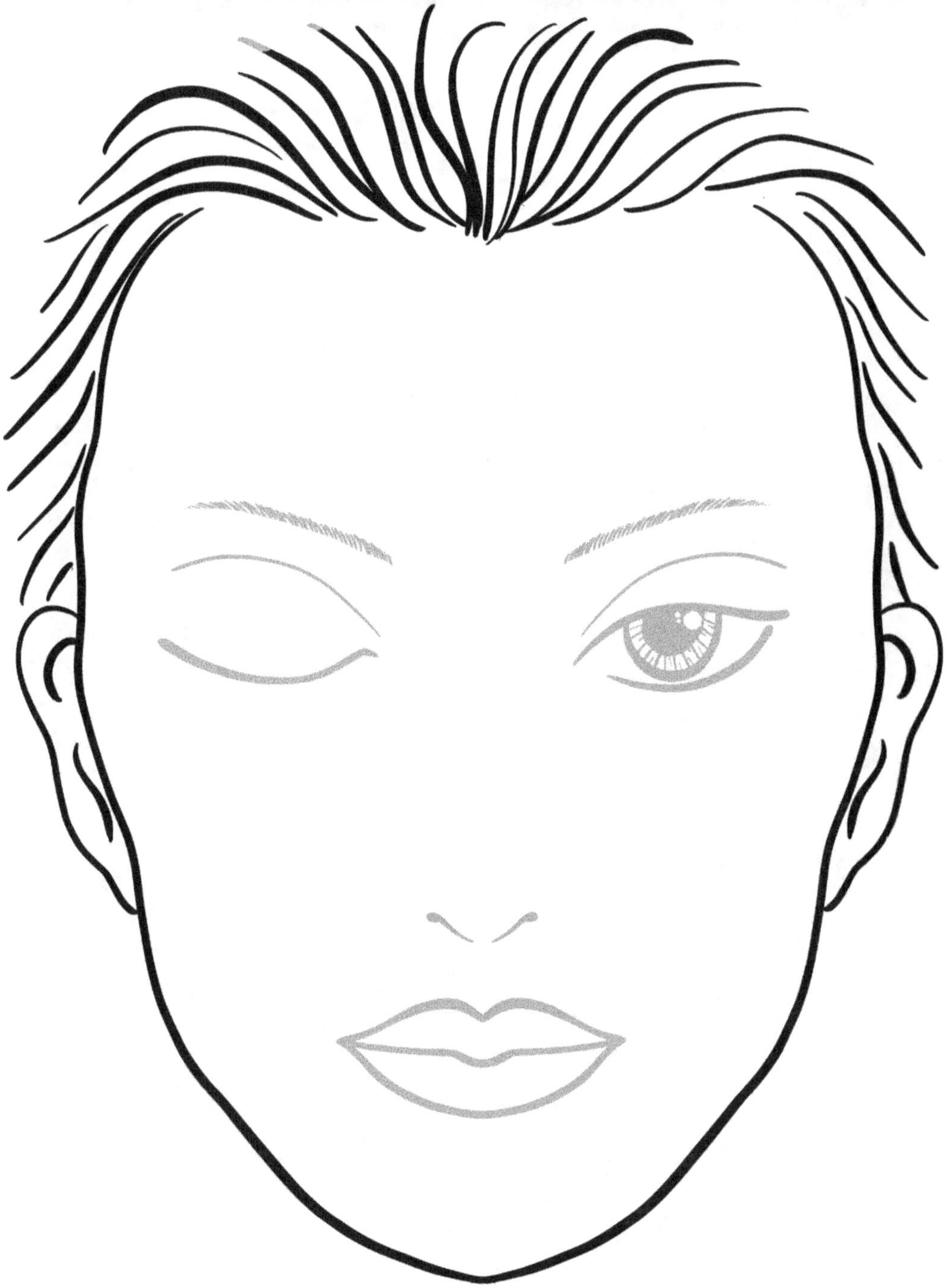

Details

Skin Tone ____________________

Eye Color ____________________

Hair Color ____________________

Lips (color, brand, etc.)

Lip Liner ____________________

Lip Color ____________________

Gloss ____________________

Eyes (color, brand, etc.)

Brows ____________________

Lid Color 1 ____________________

Lid Color 2 ____________________

Lid Color 3 ____________________

Crease ____________________

Eye Liner ____________________

Mascara ____________________

Face (color, brand, etc.)

Concealer ____________________

Foundation ____________________

Contour ____________________

Blush ____________________

Highlights ____________________

Powder ____________________

Design/Client Name ____________ Date ____________

Concealer	Foundation	Contour	Blush	Highlights	Powder	Eye Liner	Mascara
Brows	Lid Color 1	Lid Color 2	Lid Color 3	Crease	Lip Liner	Lip Color	Lip Gloss

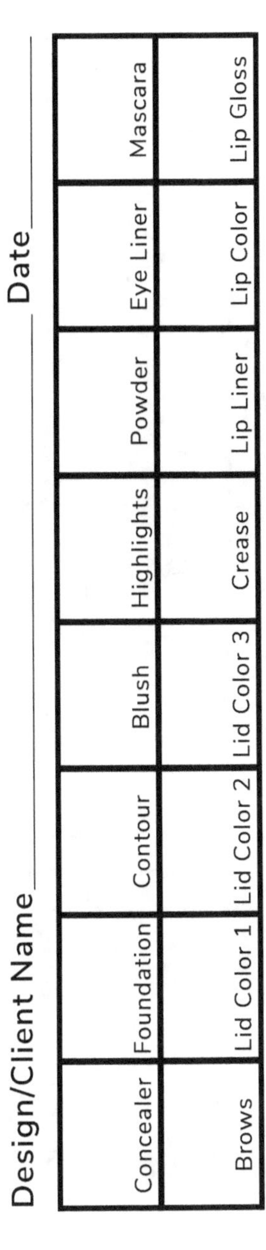

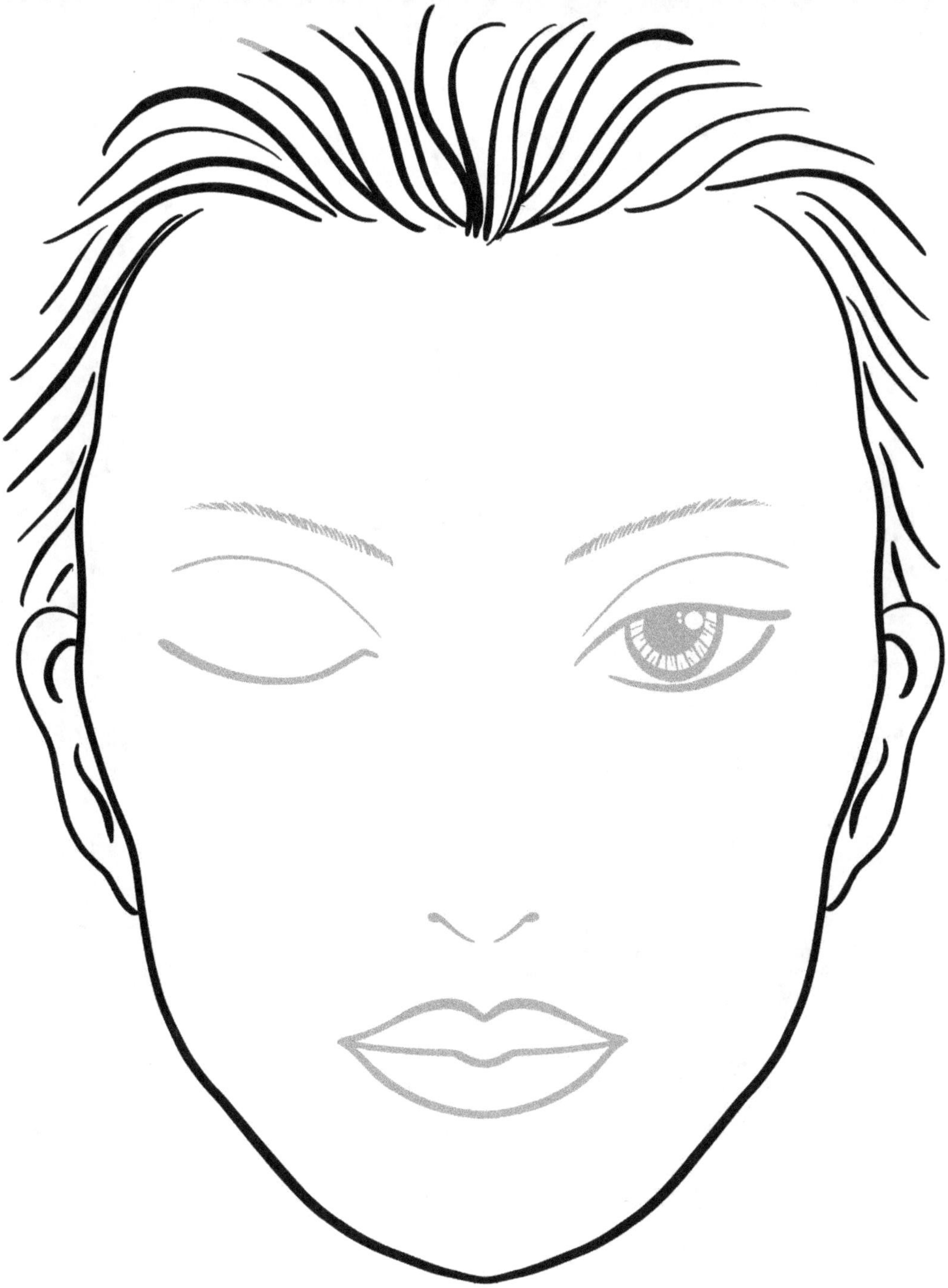

Details

Skin Tone ____________

Eye Color ____________

Hair Color ____________

Lips (color, brand, etc.)

Lip Liner ____________

Lip Color ____________

Gloss ____________

Eyes (color, brand, etc.)

Brows ____________

Lid Color 1 ____________

Lid Color 2 ____________

Lid Color 3 ____________

Crease ____________

Eye Liner ____________

Mascara ____________

Face (color, brand, etc.)

Concealer ____________

Foundation ____________

Contour ____________

Blush ____________

Highlights ____________

Powder ____________

Design/Client Name________________ Date________________

Concealer	Foundation	Contour	Blush	Highlights	Powder	Eye Liner	Mascara
Brows	Lid Color 1	Lid Color 2	Lid Color 3	Crease	Lip Liner	Lip Color	Lip Gloss

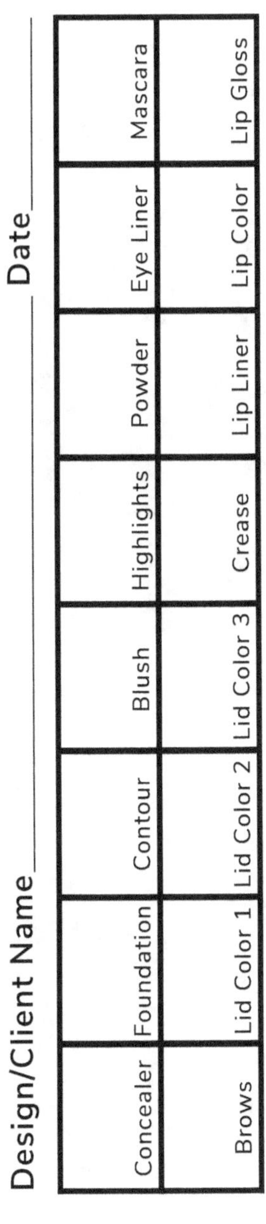

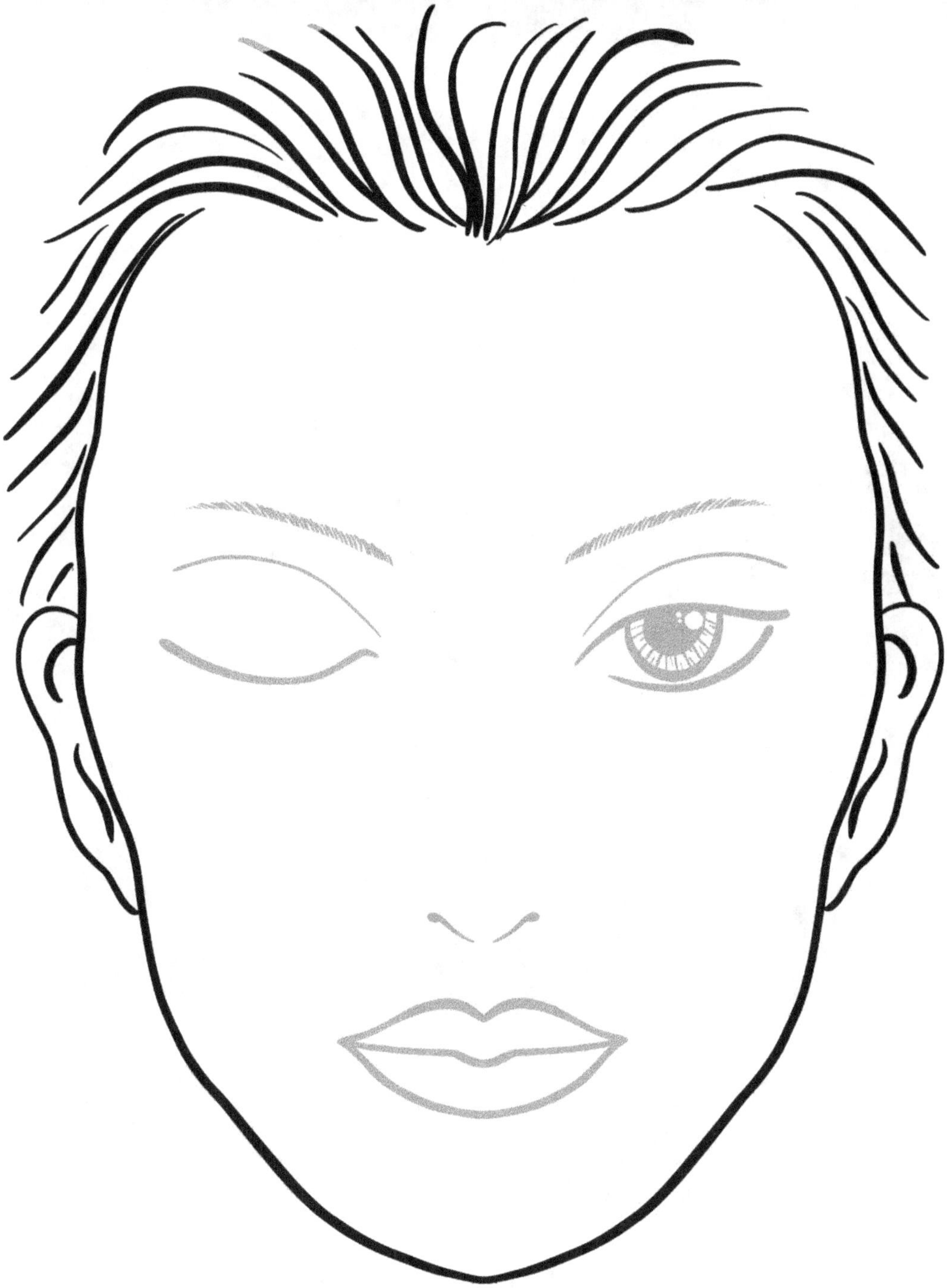

Details

Skin Tone________________

Eye Color ________________

Hair Color________________

Lips (color, brand, etc.)

Lip Liner ________________

Lip Color ________________

Gloss ________________

Eyes (color, brand, etc.)

Brows ________________

Lid Color 1 ________________

Lid Color 2 ________________

Lid Color 3 ________________

Crease________________

Eye Liner________________

Mascara ________________

Face (color, brand, etc.)

Concealer________________

Foundation________________

Contour________________

Blush ________________

Highlights ________________

Powder________________

Design/Client Name____________________ Date____________________

Concealer	Foundation	Contour	Blush	Highlights	Powder	Eye Liner	Mascara
Brows	Lid Color 1	Lid Color 2	Lid Color 3	Crease	Lip Liner	Lip Color	Lip Gloss

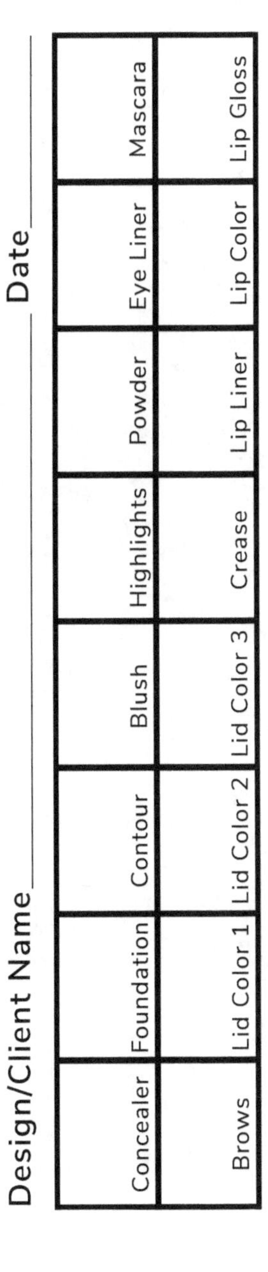

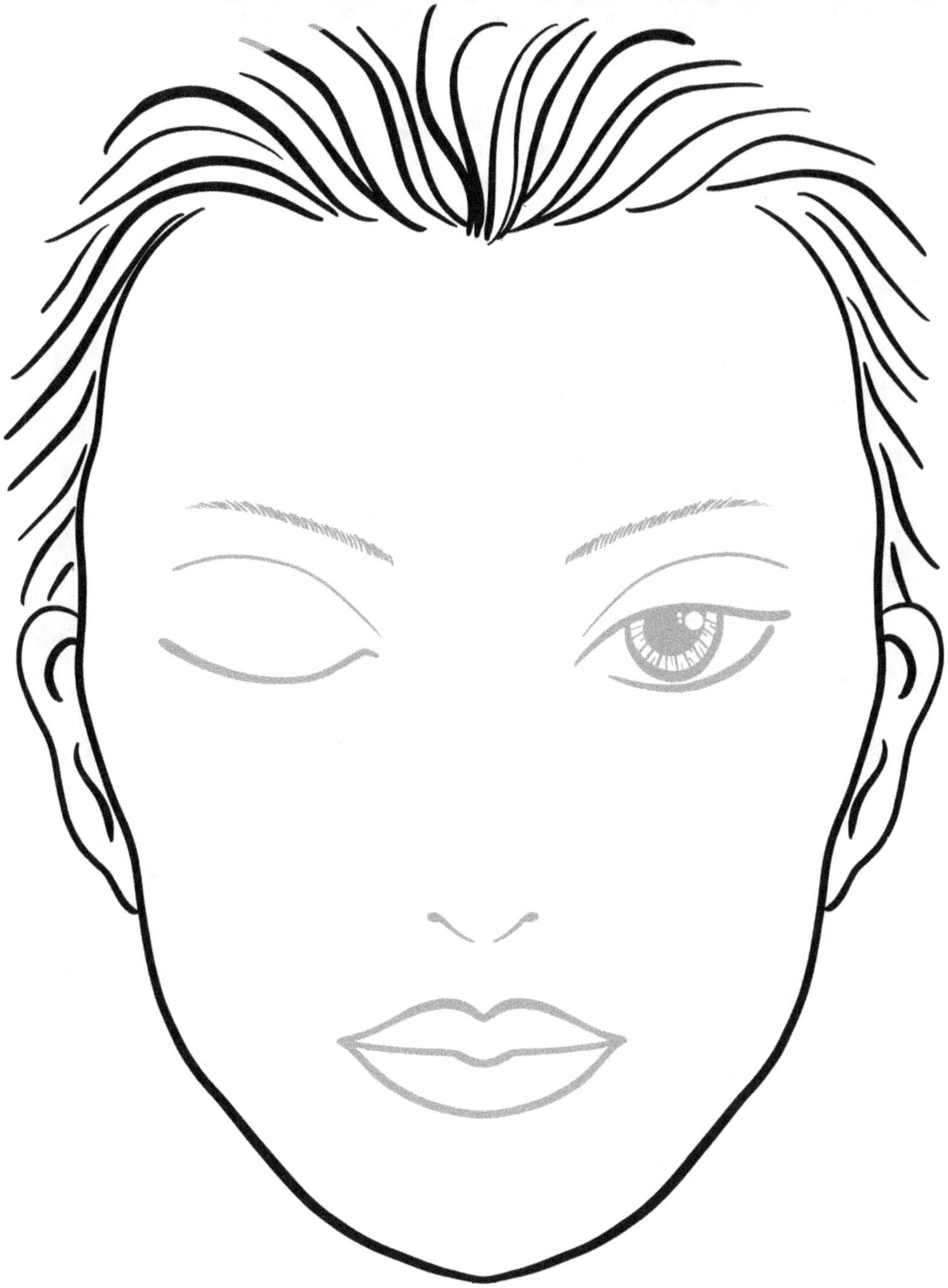

Details

Skin Tone____________________

Eye Color ____________________

Hair Color____________________

Lips (color, brand, etc.)

Lip Liner ____________________

Lip Color ____________________

Gloss ____________________

Eyes (color, brand, etc.)

Brows ____________________

Lid Color 1 ____________________

Lid Color 2 ____________________

Lid Color 3 ____________________

Crease____________________

Eye Liner____________________

Mascara ____________________

Face (color, brand, etc.)

Concealer____________________

Foundation____________________

Contour____________________

Blush ____________________

Highlights ____________________

Powder____________________

Design/Client Name____________________ Date____________

Concealer	Foundation	Contour	Blush	Highlights	Powder	Eye Liner	Mascara
Brows	Lid Color 1	Lid Color 2	Lid Color 3	Crease	Lip Liner	Lip Color	Lip Gloss

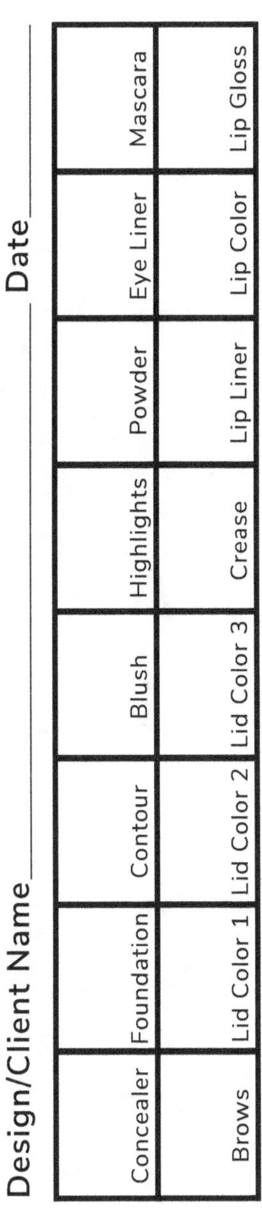

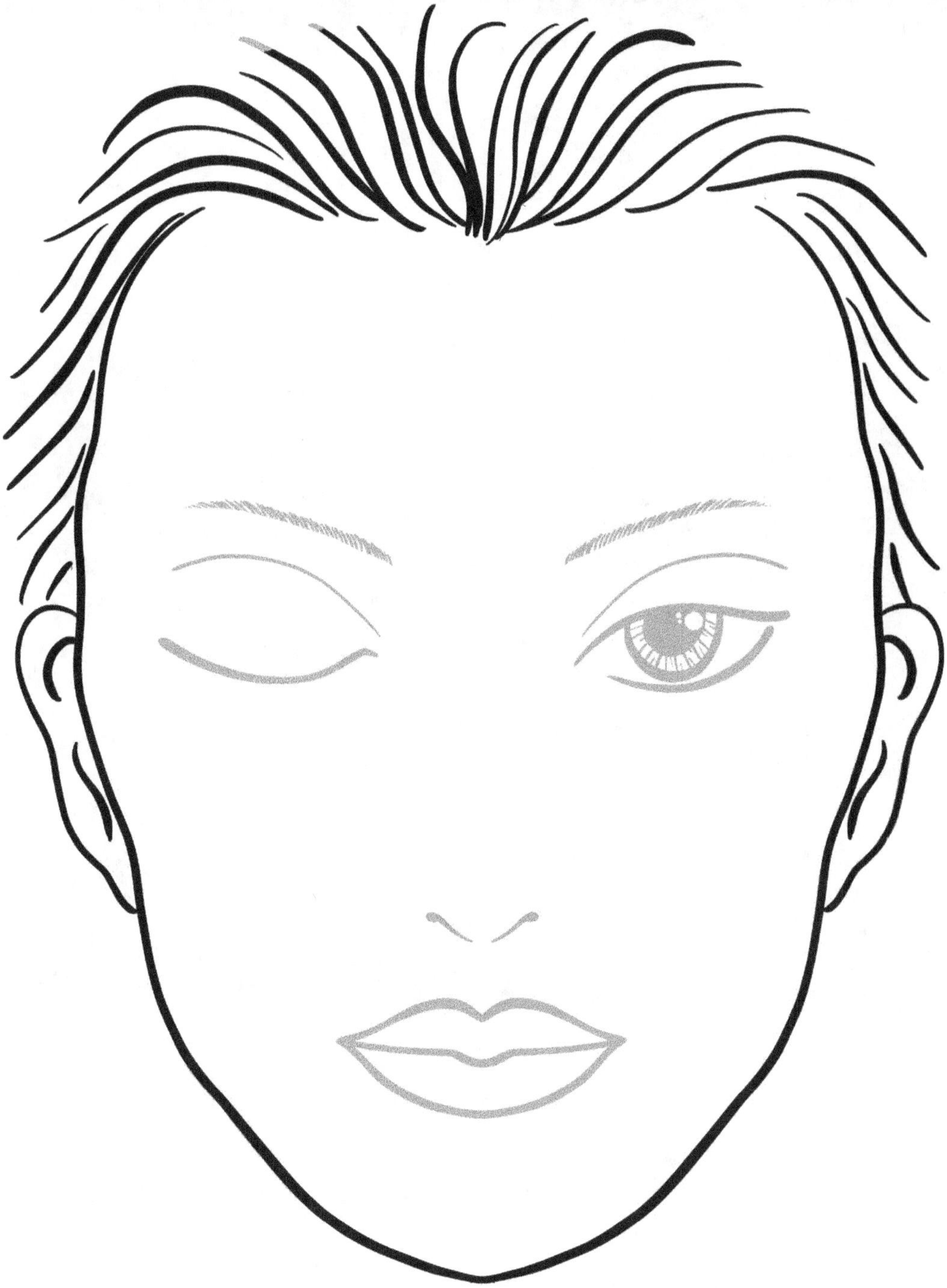

Details

Skin Tone____________________

Eye Color ____________________

Hair Color____________________

Lips (color, brand, etc.)

Lip Liner ____________________

Lip Color ____________________

Gloss ____________________

Eyes (color, brand, etc.)

Brows ____________________

Lid Color 1 ____________________

Lid Color 2 ____________________

Lid Color 3 ____________________

Crease____________________

Eye Liner____________________

Mascara ____________________

Face (color, brand, etc.)

Concealer____________________

Foundation____________________

Contour____________________

Blush ____________________

Highlights ____________________

Powder____________________

Design/Client Name ____________________ Date ____________________

Concealer	Foundation	Contour	Blush	Highlights	Powder	Eye Liner	Mascara
Brows	Lid Color 1	Lid Color 2	Lid Color 3	Crease	Lip Liner	Lip Color	Lip Gloss

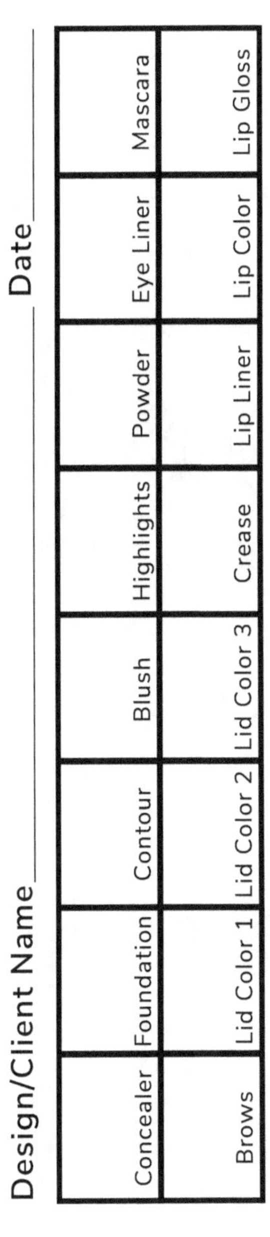

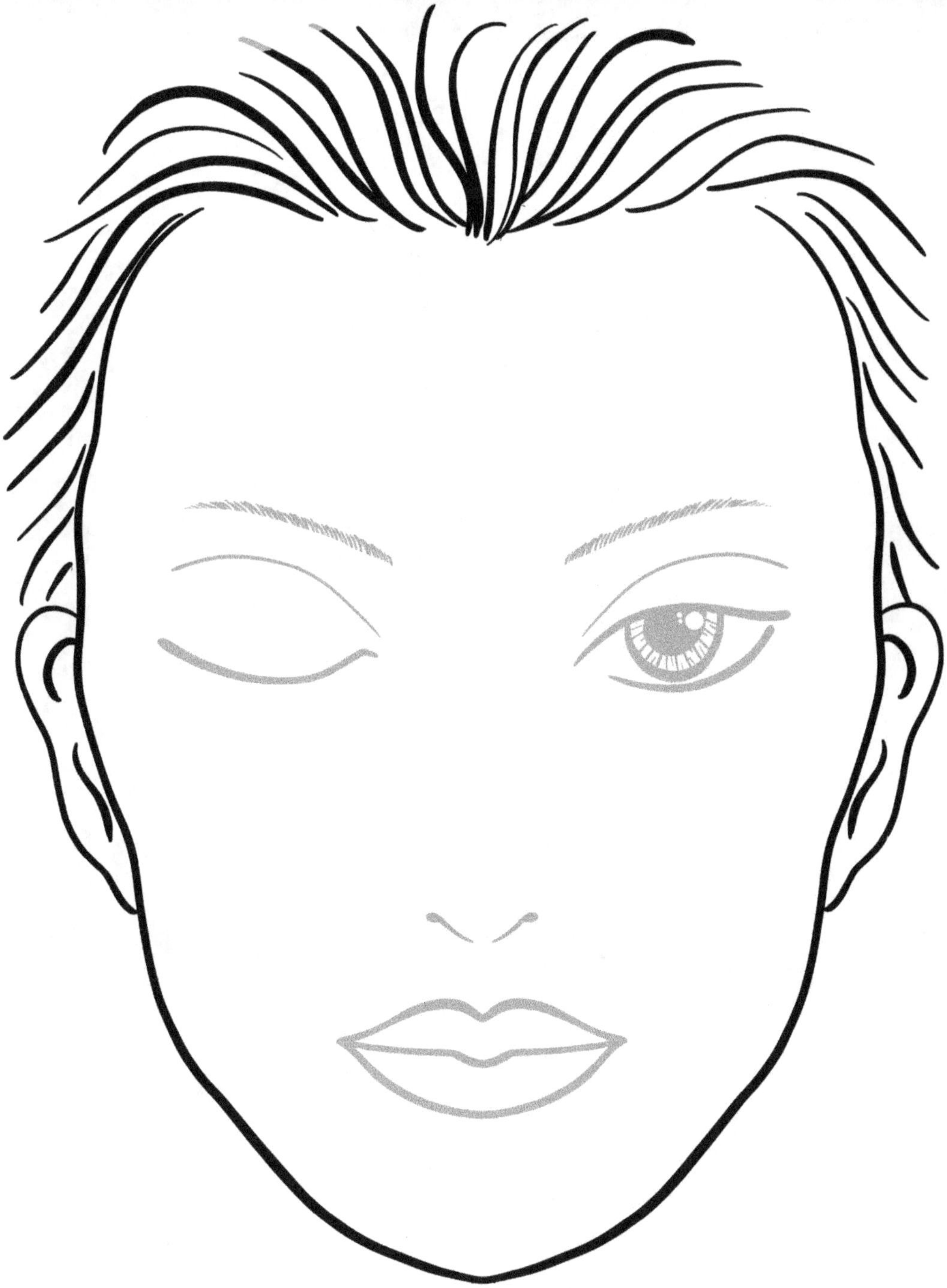

Details

Skin Tone ____________________

Eye Color ____________________

Hair Color ____________________

Lips (color, brand, etc.)

Lip Liner ____________________

Lip Color ____________________

Gloss ____________________

Eyes (color, brand, etc.)

Brows ____________________

Lid Color 1 ____________________

Lid Color 2 ____________________

Lid Color 3 ____________________

Crease ____________________

Eye Liner ____________________

Mascara ____________________

Face (color, brand, etc.)

Concealer ____________________

Foundation ____________________

Contour ____________________

Blush ____________________

Highlights ____________________

Powder ____________________

Design/Client Name________________ Date________________

Concealer	Foundation	Contour	Blush	Highlights	Powder	Eye Liner	Mascara
Brows	Lid Color 1	Lid Color 2	Lid Color 3	Crease	Lip Liner	Lip Color	Lip Gloss

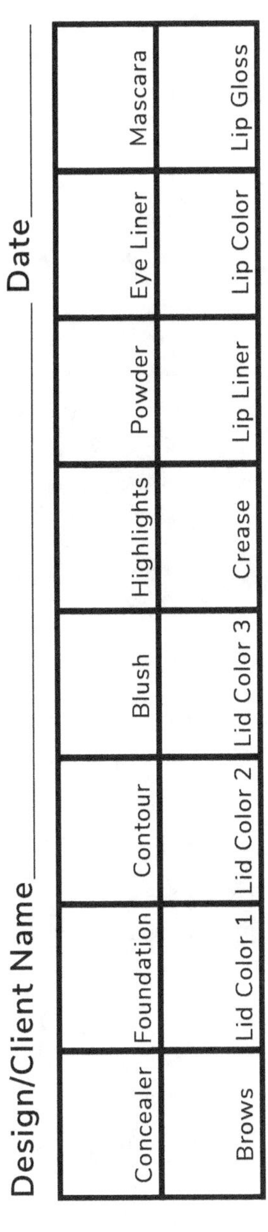

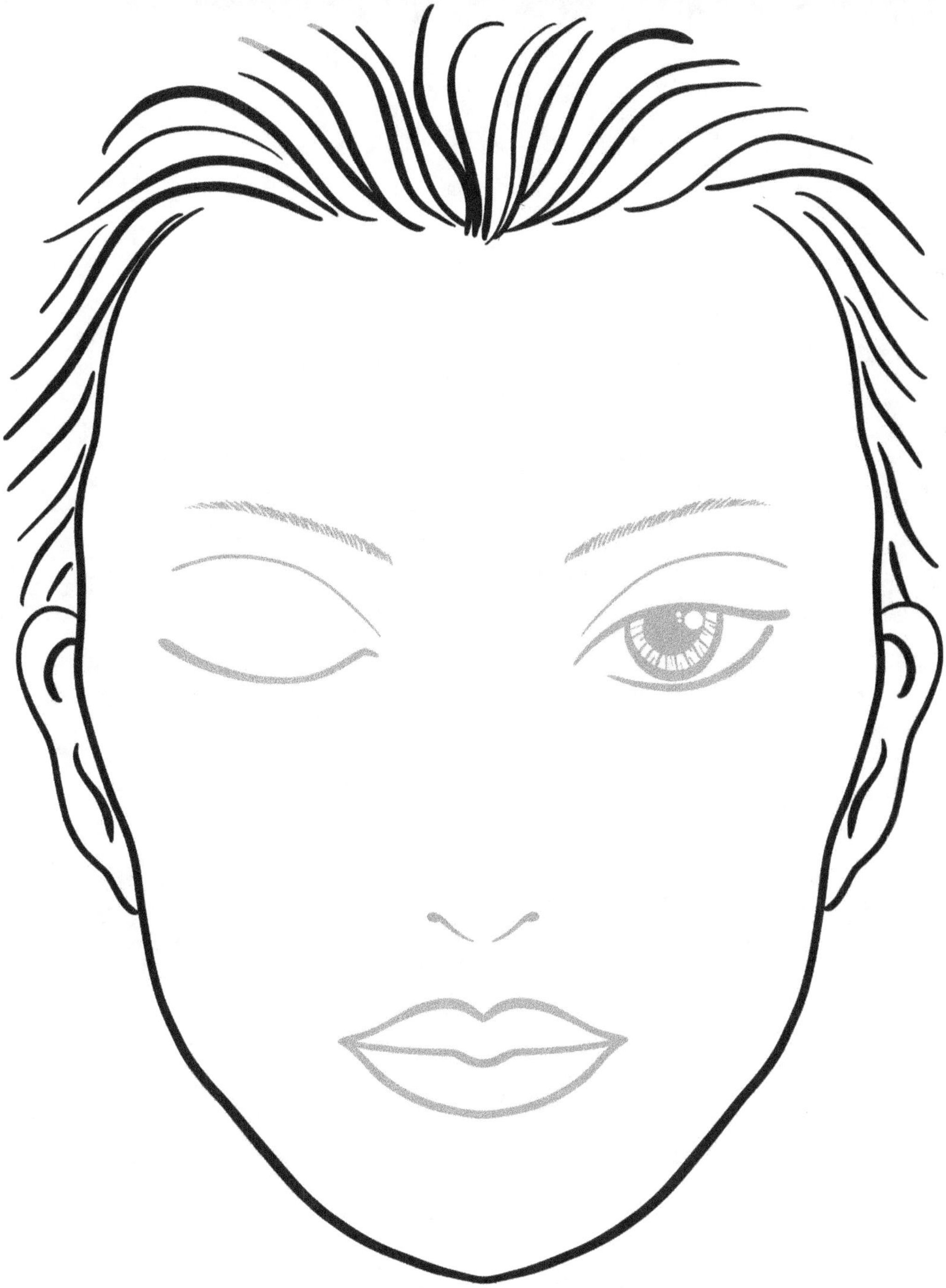

Details

Skin Tone________________

Eye Color ________________

Hair Color________________

Lips (color, brand, etc.)

Lip Liner ________________

Lip Color ________________

Gloss ________________

Eyes (color, brand, etc.)

Brows ________________

Lid Color 1 ________________

Lid Color 2 ________________

Lid Color 3 ________________

Crease________________

Eye Liner________________

Mascara ________________

Face (color, brand, etc.)

Concealer________________

Foundation________________

Contour________________

Blush ________________

Highlights ________________

Powder________________

Design/Client Name________________ Date________

Concealer	Foundation	Contour	Blush	Highlights	Powder	Eye Liner	Mascara
Brows	Lid Color 1	Lid Color 2	Lid Color 3	Crease	Lip Liner	Lip Color	Lip Gloss

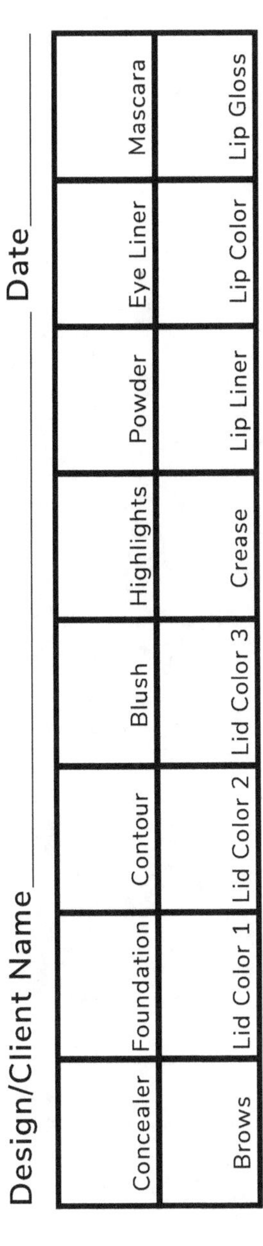

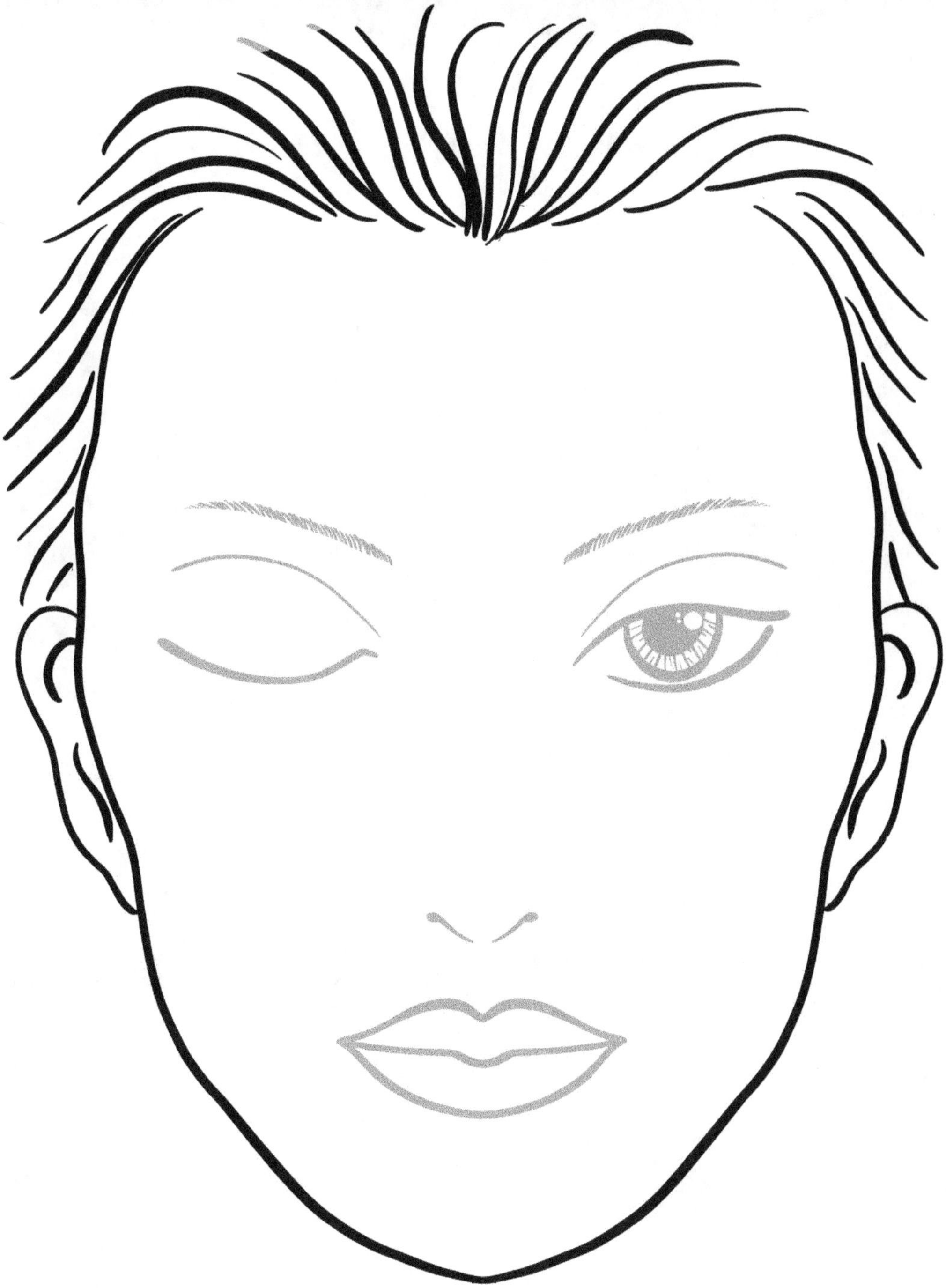

Details

Skin Tone____________________

Eye Color ____________________

Hair Color____________________

Lips (color, brand, etc.)

Lip Liner ____________________

Lip Color ____________________

Gloss ____________________

Eyes (color, brand, etc.)

Brows ________________________

Lid Color 1 ____________________

Lid Color 2 ____________________

Lid Color 3 ____________________

Crease ________________________

Eye Liner______________________

Mascara ______________________

Face (color, brand, etc.)

Concealer____________________

Foundation___________________

Contour______________________

Blush ______________________

Highlights ___________________

Powder______________________

Design/Client Name________________ Date________________

Concealer	Brows
Foundation	Lid Color 1
Contour	Lid Color 2
Blush	Lid Color 3
Highlights	Crease
Powder	Lip Liner
Eye Liner	Lip Color
Mascara	Lip Gloss

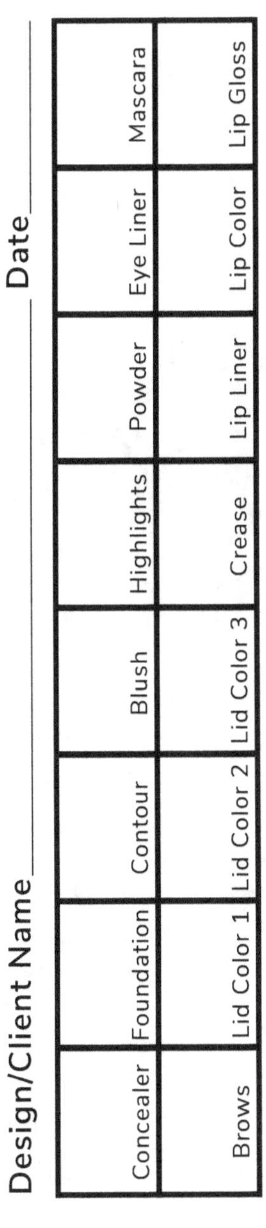

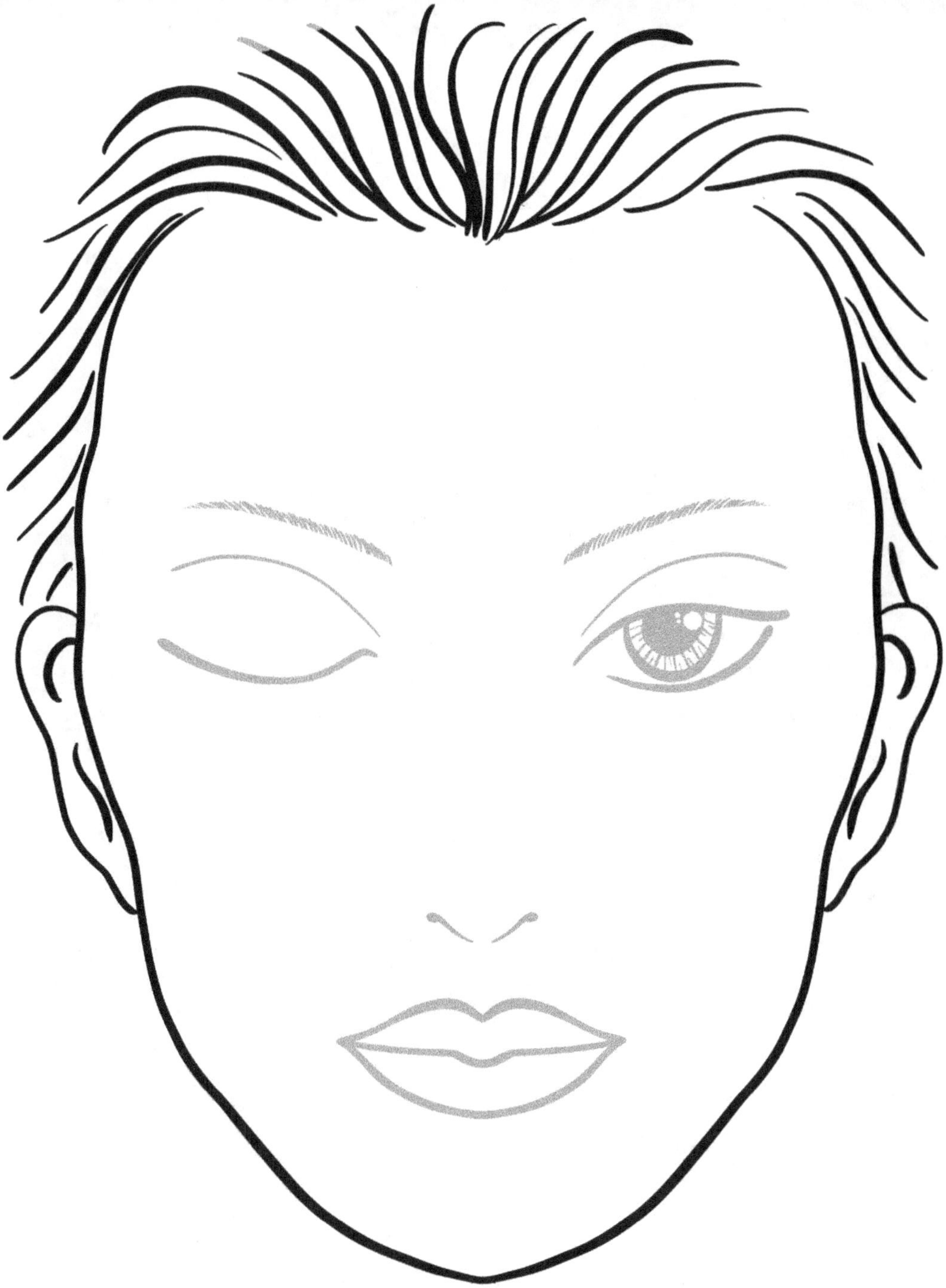

Details

Skin Tone________________

Eye Color ________________

Hair Color________________

Lips (color, brand, etc.)

Lip Liner ________________

Lip Color ________________

Gloss ________________

Eyes (color, brand, etc.)

Brows ________________

Lid Color 1 ________________

Lid Color 2 ________________

Lid Color 3 ________________

Crease________________

Eye Liner________________

Mascara ________________

Face (color, brand, etc.)

Concealer________________

Foundation________________

Contour________________

Blush ________________

Highlights ________________

Powder________________

Design/Client Name ______________________ Date ______________

Concealer	Foundation	Contour	Blush	Highlights	Powder	Eye Liner	Mascara
Brows	Lid Color 1	Lid Color 2	Lid Color 3	Crease	Lip Liner	Lip Color	Lip Gloss

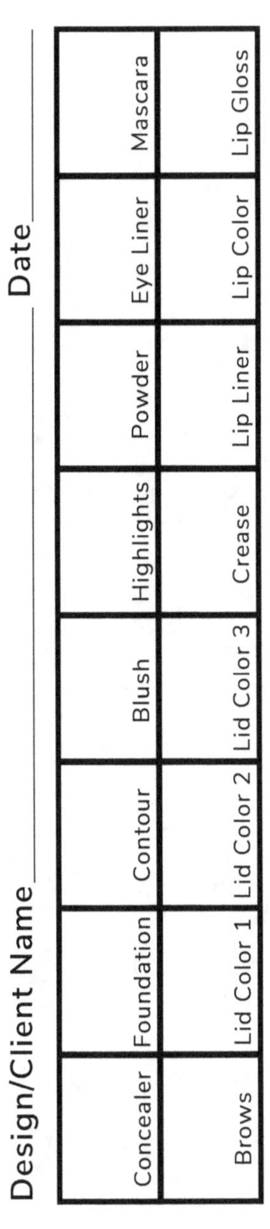

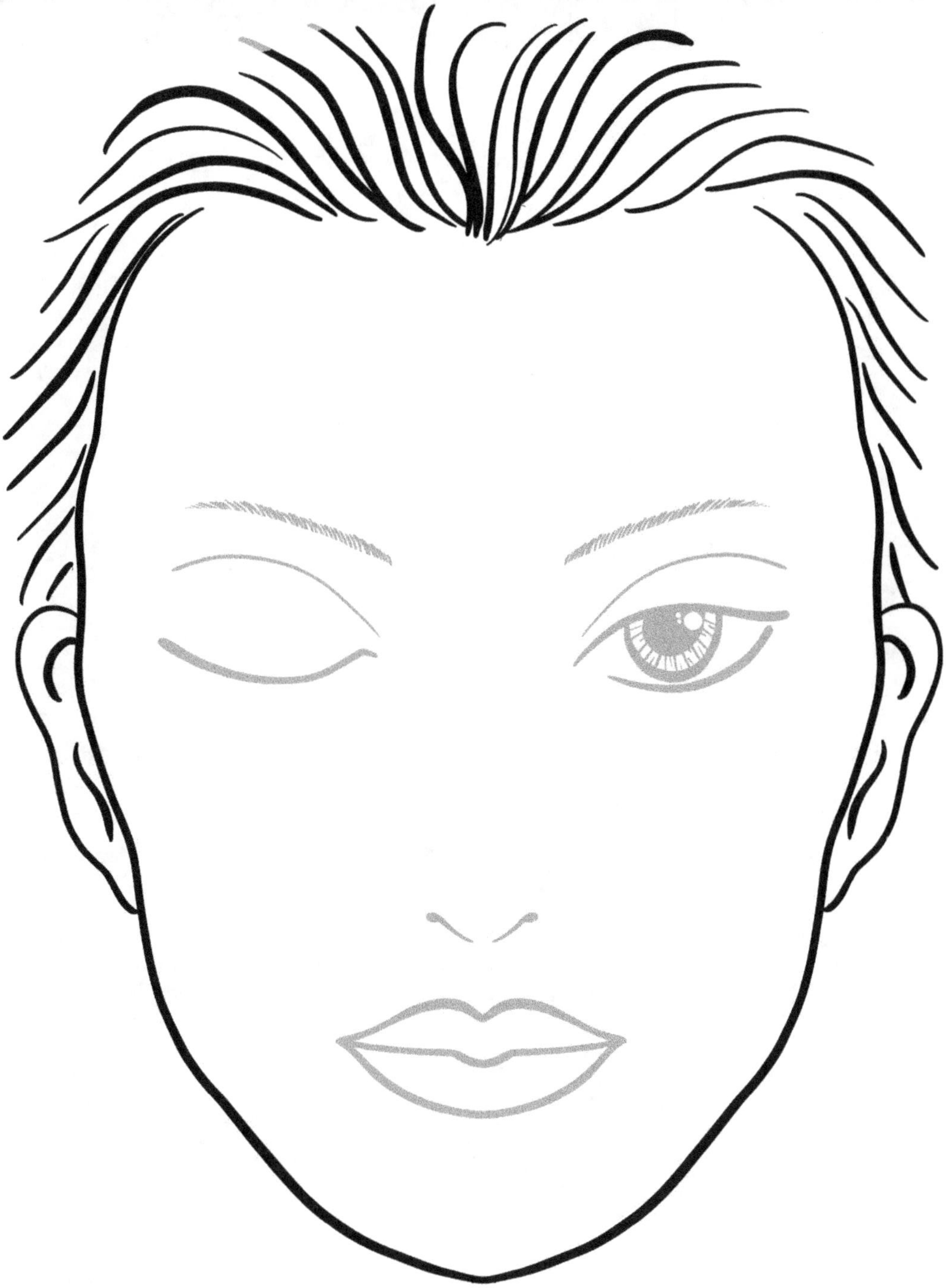

Details

Skin Tone ____________________

Eye Color ____________________

Hair Color ____________________

Lips (color, brand, etc.)

Lip Liner ____________________

Lip Color ____________________

Gloss ____________________

Eyes (color, brand, etc.)

Brows ____________________

Lid Color 1 ____________________

Lid Color 2 ____________________

Lid Color 3 ____________________

Crease ____________________

Eye Liner ____________________

Mascara ____________________

Face (color, brand, etc.)

Concealer ____________________

Foundation ____________________

Contour ____________________

Blush ____________________

Highlights ____________________

Powder ____________________

Design/Client Name__________________ Date__________

Concealer	Foundation	Contour	Blush	Highlights	Powder	Eye Liner	Mascara
Brows	Lid Color 1	Lid Color 2	Lid Color 3	Crease	Lip Liner	Lip Color	Lip Gloss

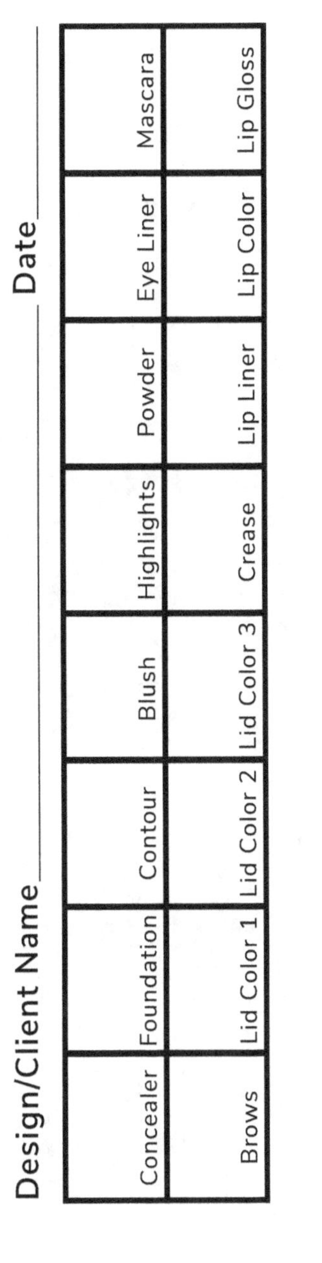

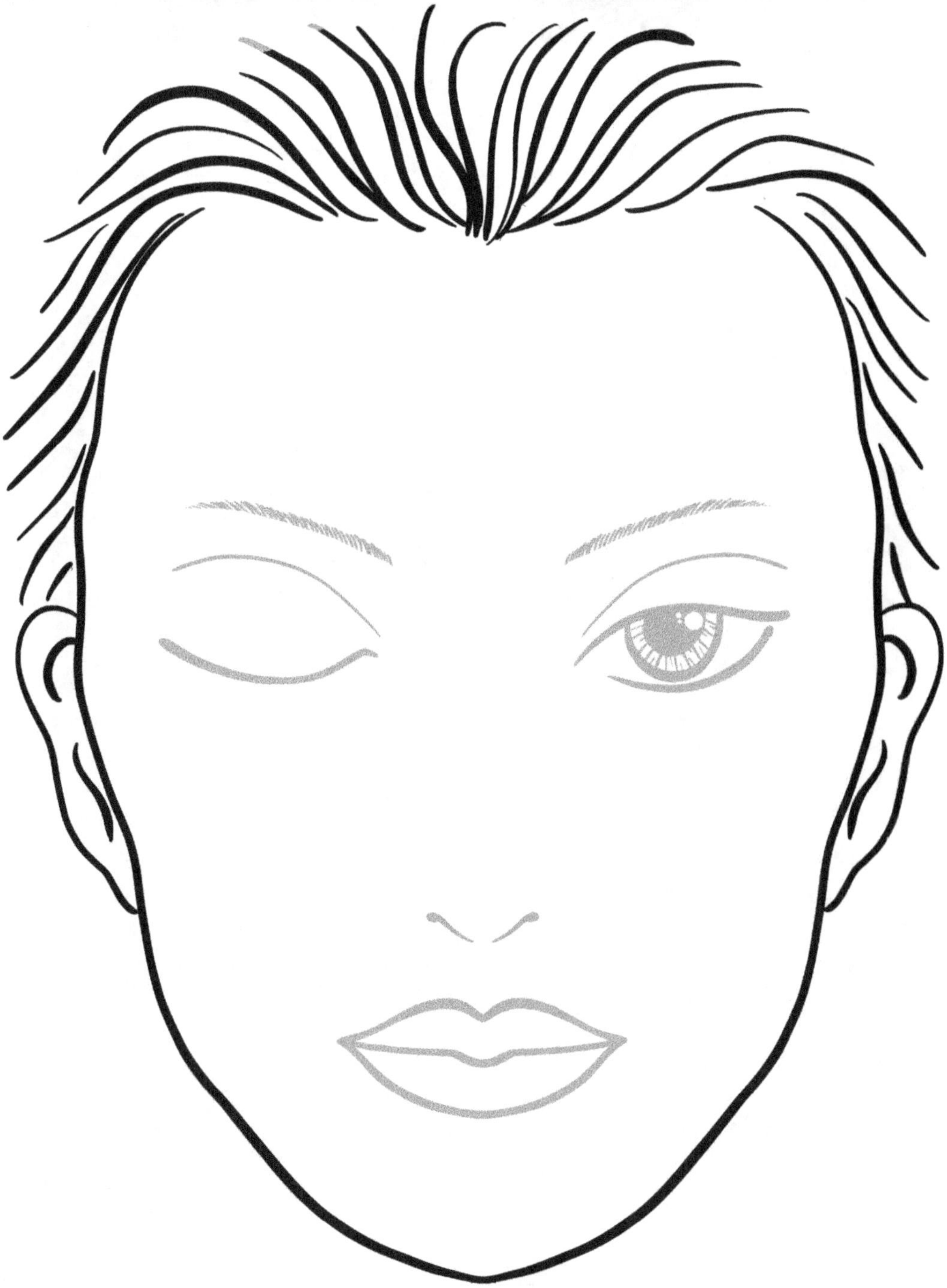

Details

Skin Tone____________________

Eye Color ____________________

Hair Color____________________

Lips (color, brand, etc.)

Lip Liner ____________________

Lip Color ____________________

Gloss ____________________

Eyes (color, brand, etc.)

Brows ____________________

Lid Color 1 ____________________

Lid Color 2 ____________________

Lid Color 3 ____________________

Crease ____________________

Eye Liner____________________

Mascara ____________________

Face (color, brand, etc.)

Concealer____________________

Foundation____________________

Contour____________________

Blush ____________________

Highlights ____________________

Powder____________________

Design/Client Name____________ Date____________

Concealer	Foundation	Contour	Blush	Highlights	Powder	Eye Liner	Mascara
Brows	Lid Color 1	Lid Color 2	Lid Color 3	Crease	Lip Liner	Lip Color	Lip Gloss

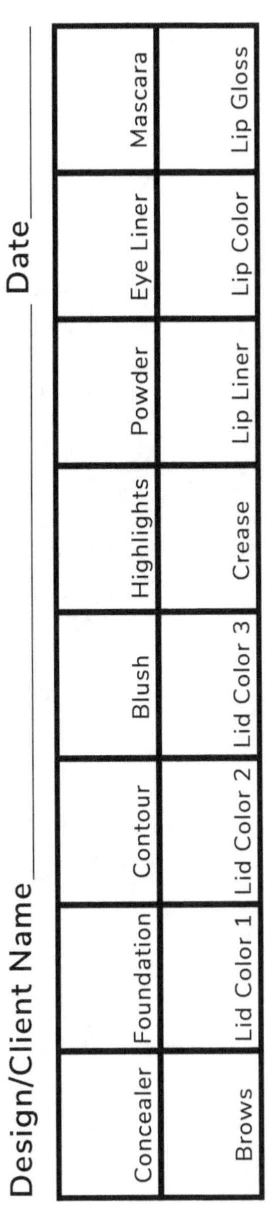

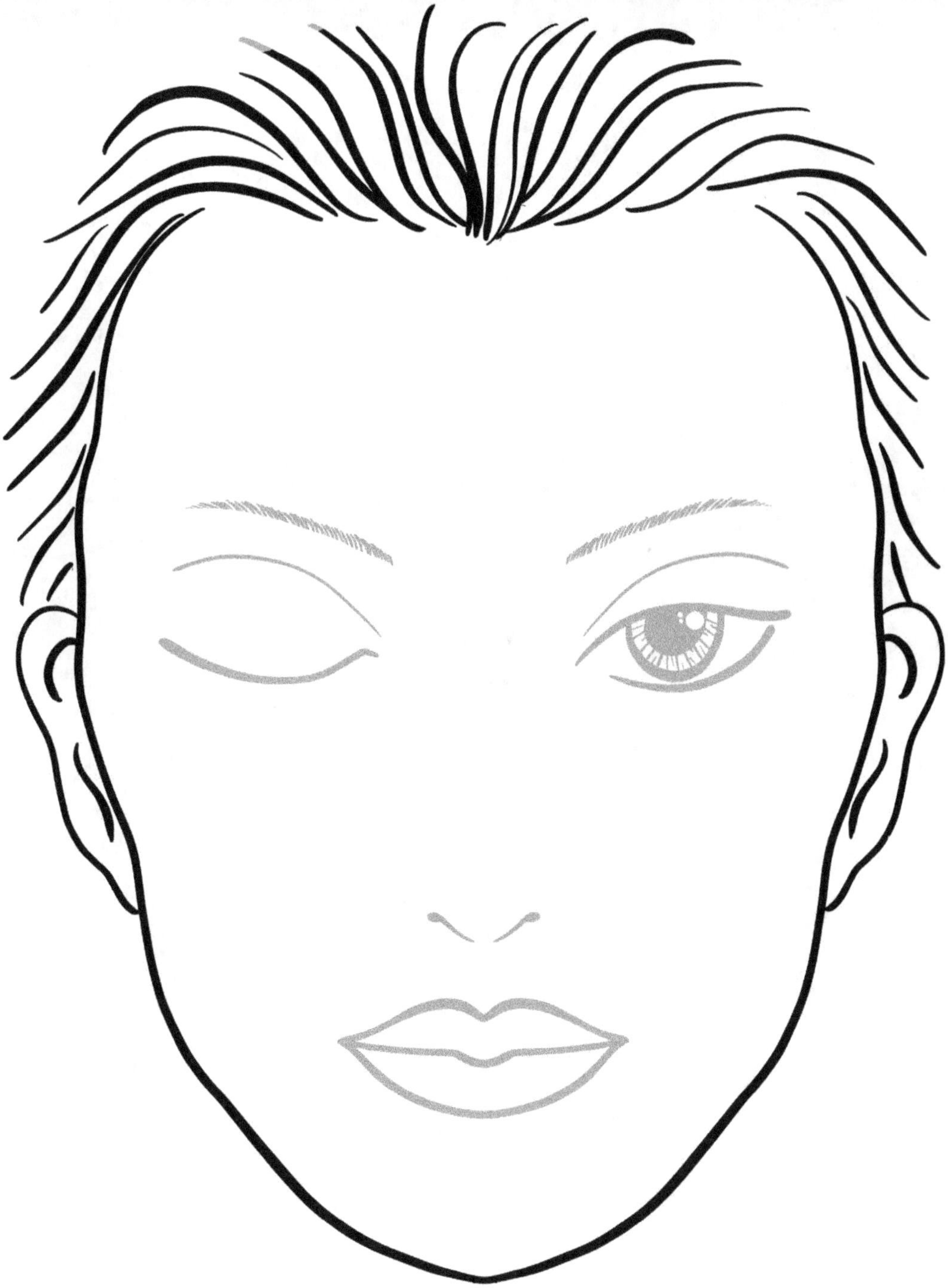

Details

Skin Tone____________________

Eye Color ____________________

Hair Color____________________

Lips (color, brand, etc.)

Lip Liner ____________________

Lip Color ____________________

Gloss ____________________

Eyes (color, brand, etc.)

Brows ____________________

Lid Color 1 ____________________

Lid Color 2 ____________________

Lid Color 3 ____________________

Crease____________________

Eye Liner____________________

Mascara ____________________

Face (color, brand, etc.)

Concealer____________________

Foundation____________________

Contour____________________

Blush ____________________

Highlights ____________________

Powder____________________

Design/Client Name ____________ Date ____________

Concealer	Foundation	Contour	Blush	Highlights	Powder	Eye Liner	Mascara
Brows	Lid Color 1	Lid Color 2	Lid Color 3	Crease	Lip Liner	Lip Color	Lip Gloss

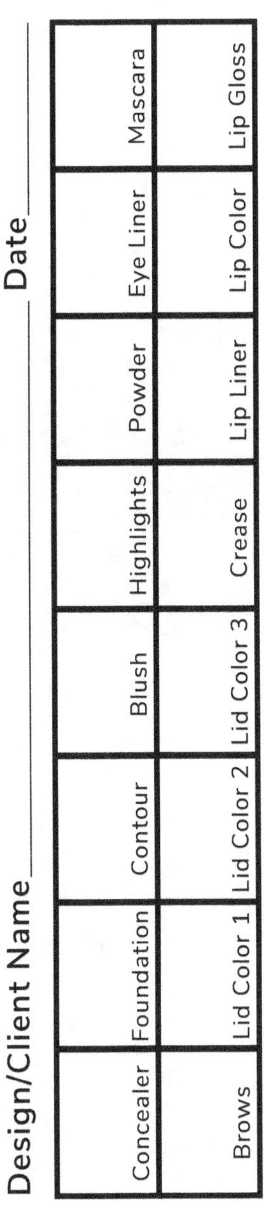

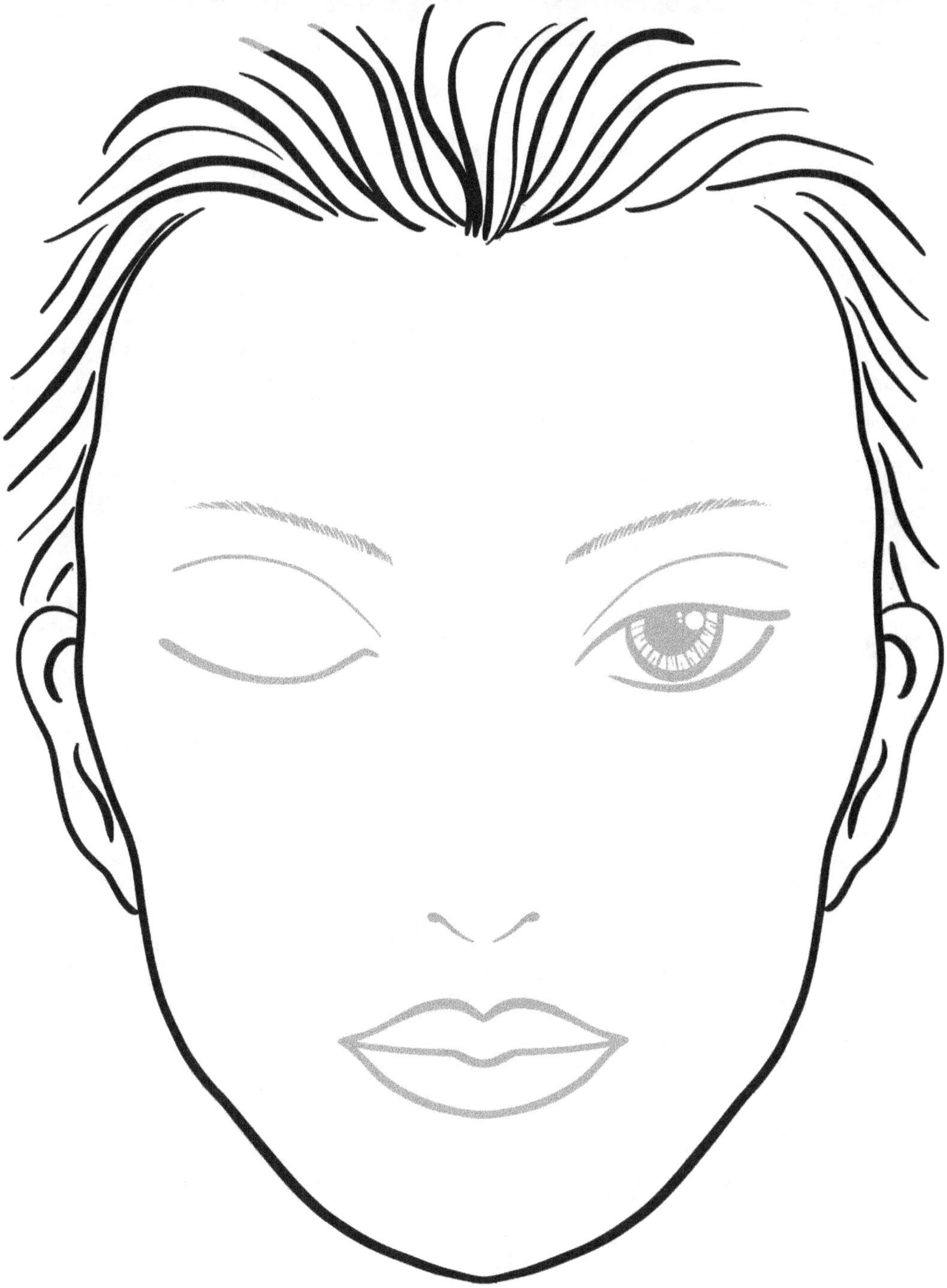

Details

Skin Tone ____________________

Eye Color ____________________

Hair Color ____________________

Lips (color, brand, etc.)

Lip Liner ____________________

Lip Color ____________________

Gloss ____________________

Eyes (color, brand, etc.)

Brows ____________________

Lid Color 1 ____________________

Lid Color 2 ____________________

Lid Color 3 ____________________

Crease ____________________

Eye Liner ____________________

Mascara ____________________

Face (color, brand, etc.)

Concealer ____________________

Foundation ____________________

Contour ____________________

Blush ____________________

Highlights ____________________

Powder ____________________

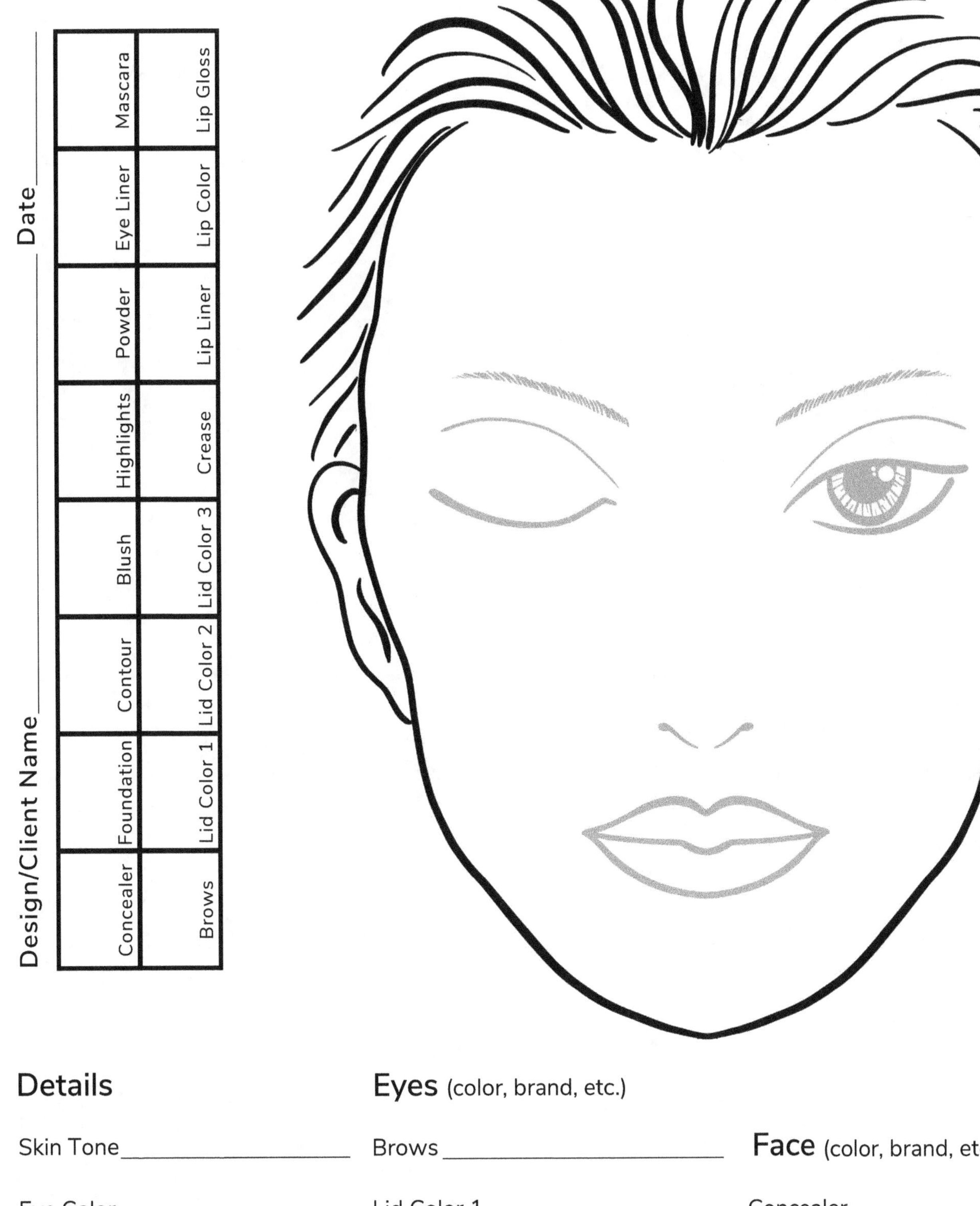

Details

Skin Tone _______________________

Eye Color _______________________

Hair Color _______________________

Lips (color, brand, etc.)

Lip Liner _______________________

Lip Color _______________________

Gloss _______________________

Eyes (color, brand, etc.)

Brows _______________________

Lid Color 1 _______________________

Lid Color 2 _______________________

Lid Color 3 _______________________

Crease _______________________

Eye Liner _______________________

Mascara _______________________

Face (color, brand, etc.)

Concealer _______________________

Foundation _______________________

Contour _______________________

Blush _______________________

Highlights _______________________

Powder _______________________

Design/Client Name____________________ Date____________________

Concealer	Brows
Foundation	Lid Color 1
Contour	Lid Color 2
Blush	Lid Color 3
Highlights	Crease
Powder	Lip Liner
Eye Liner	Lip Color
Mascara	Lip Gloss

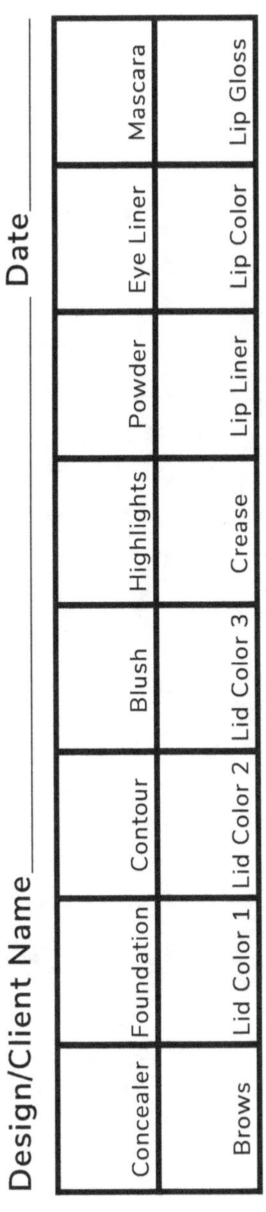

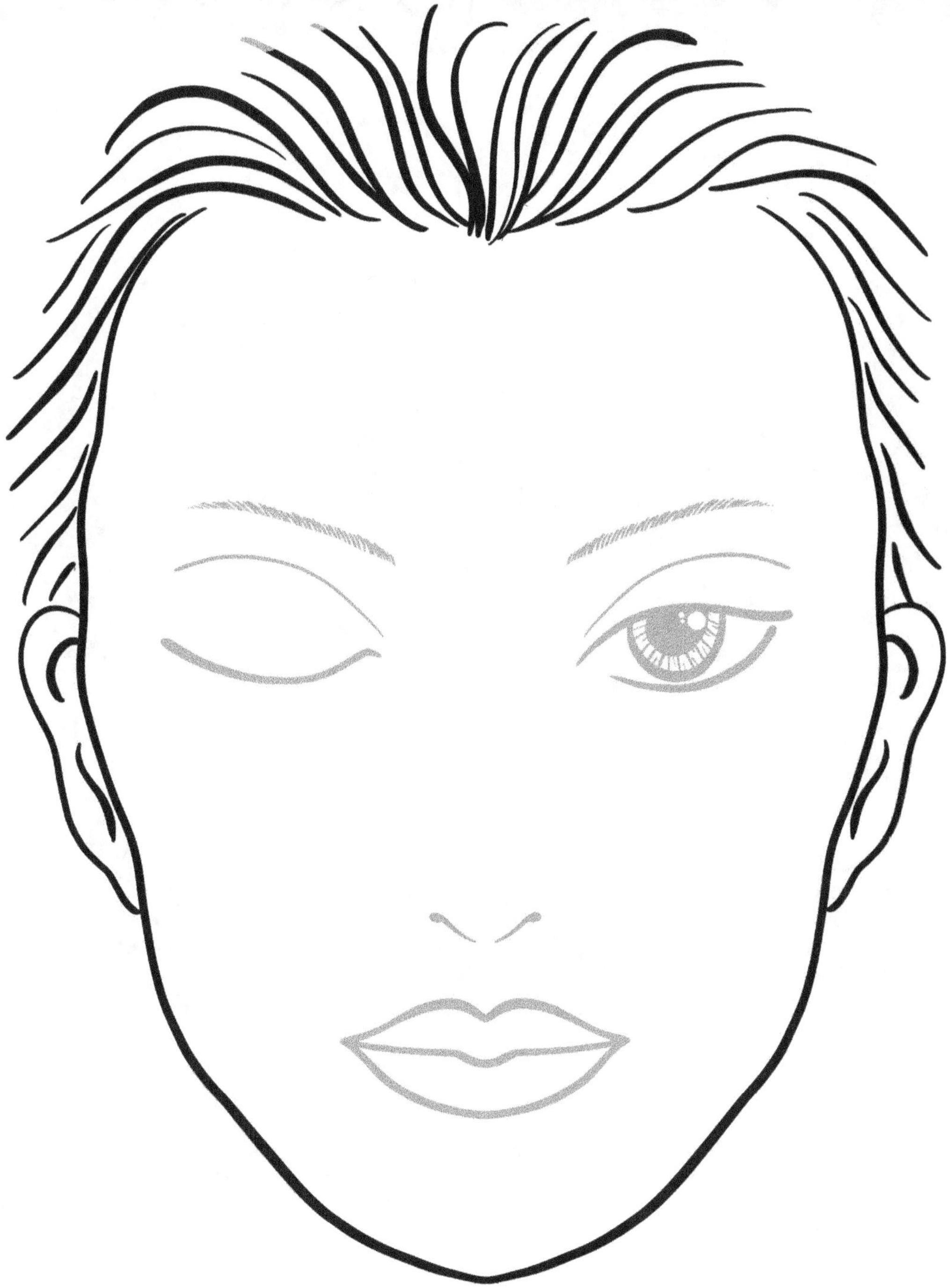

Details

Skin Tone____________________

Eye Color ____________________

Hair Color____________________

Lips (color, brand, etc.)

Lip Liner ____________________

Lip Color ____________________

Gloss ____________________

Eyes (color, brand, etc.)

Brows ____________________

Lid Color 1 ____________________

Lid Color 2 ____________________

Lid Color 3 ____________________

Crease____________________

Eye Liner____________________

Mascara ____________________

Face (color, brand, etc.)

Concealer____________________

Foundation____________________

Contour____________________

Blush ____________________

Highlights ____________________

Powder____________________

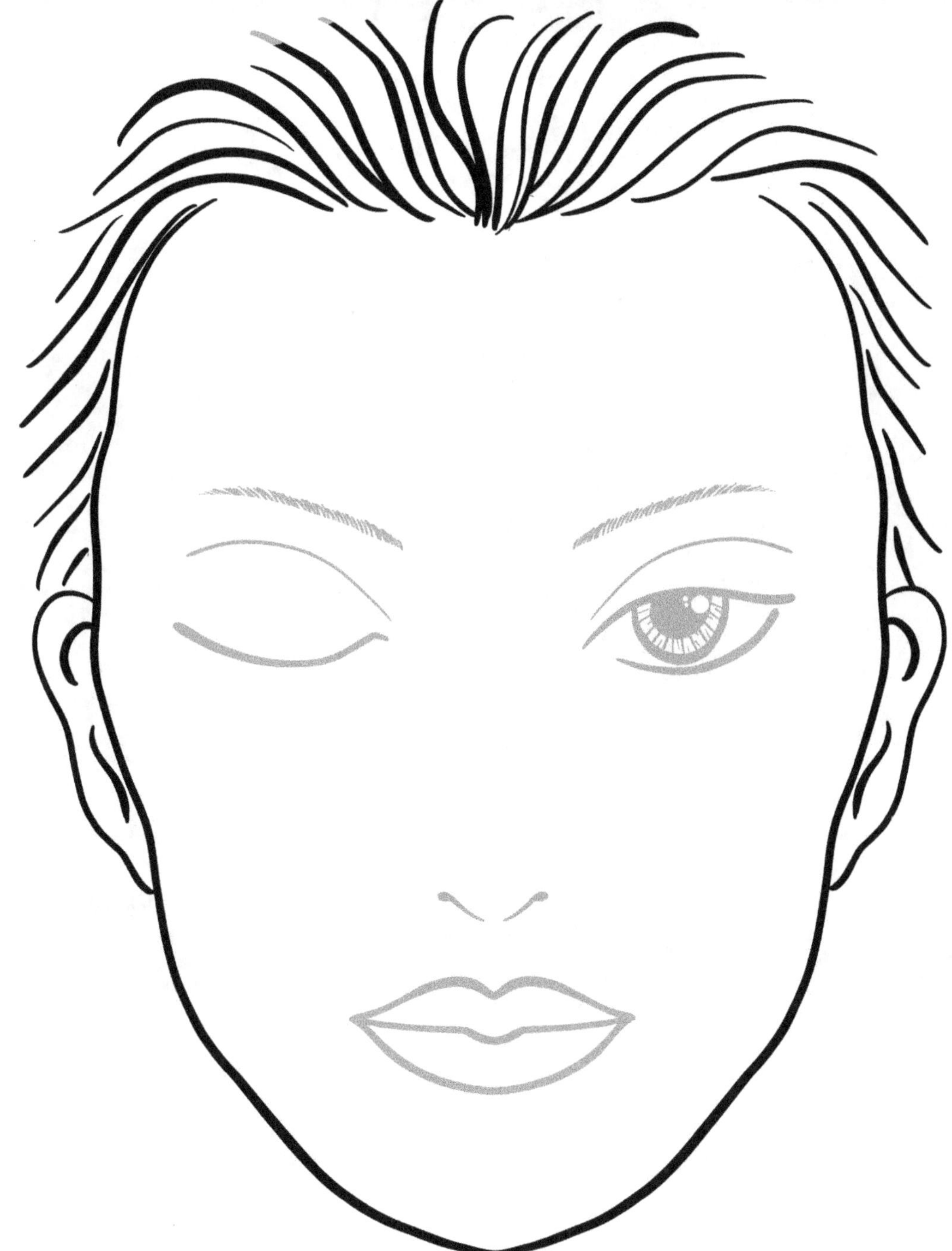

Details

Skin Tone____________________

Eye Color ___________________

Hair Color__________________

Lips (color, brand, etc.)

Lip Liner _________________

Lip Color _________________

Gloss ____________________

Eyes (color, brand, etc.)

Brows ___________________

Lid Color 1 ________________

Lid Color 2 ________________

Lid Color 3 ________________

Crease __________________

Eye Liner_________________

Mascara _________________

Face (color, brand, etc.)

Concealer_________________

Foundation________________

Contour__________________

Blush ___________________

Highlights _______________

Powder__________________

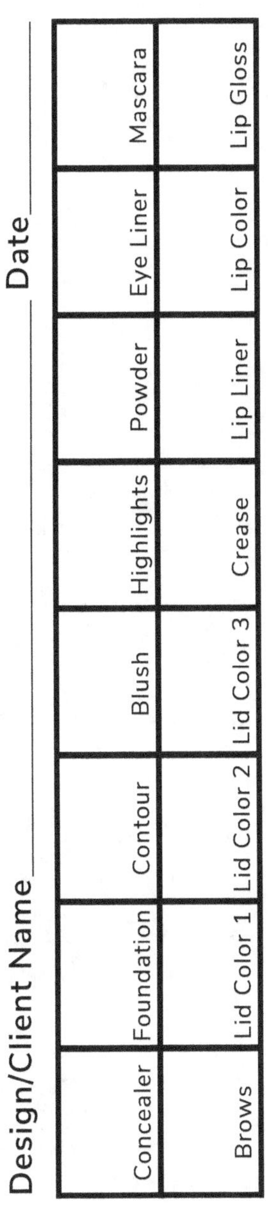

Design/Client Name____________________ Date_______________

Concealer	Foundation	Contour	Blush	Highlights	Powder	Eye Liner	Mascara
Brows	Lid Color 1	Lid Color 2	Lid Color 3	Crease	Lip Liner	Lip Color	Lip Gloss

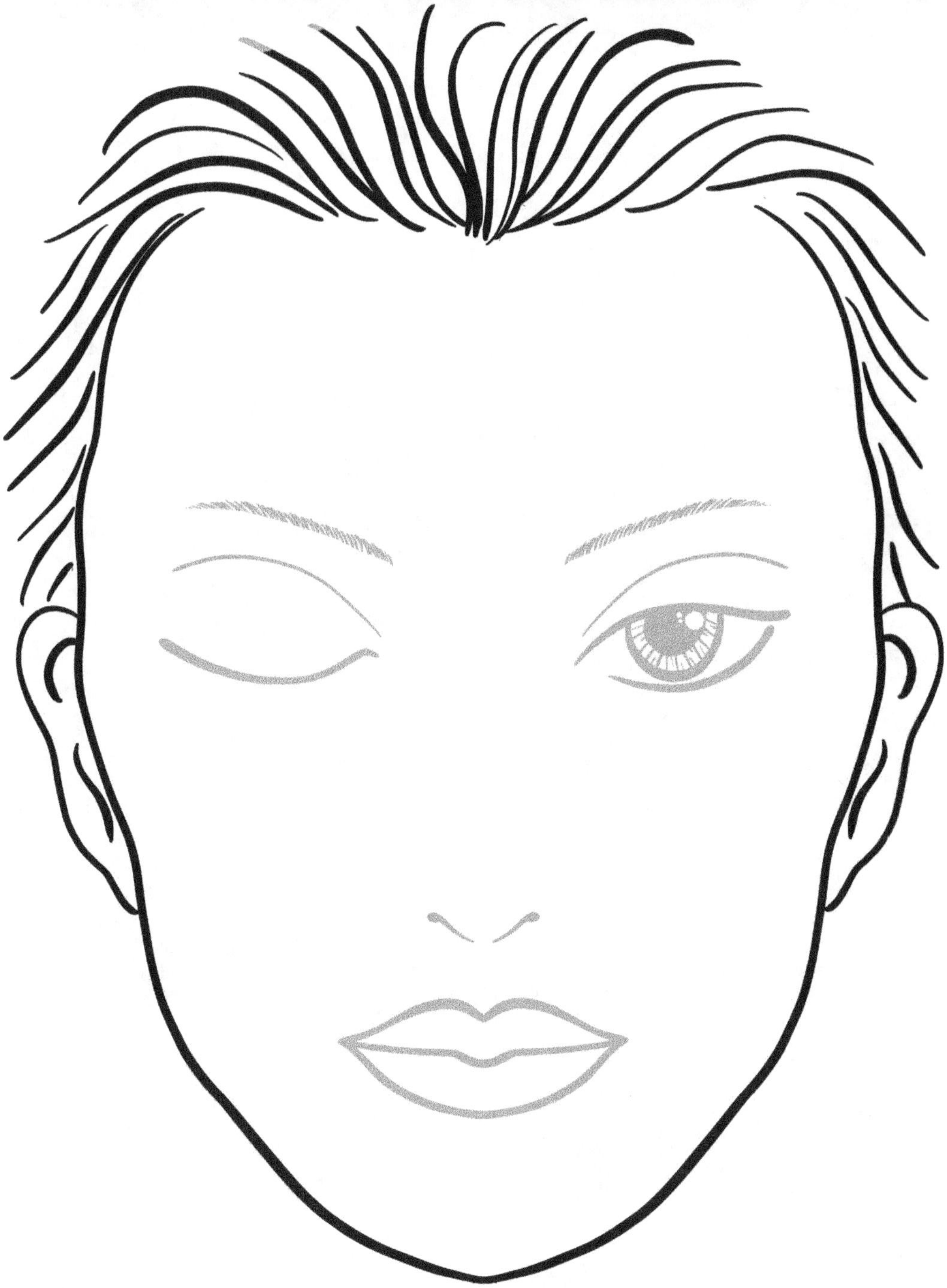

Details

Skin Tone____________________

Eye Color ____________________

Hair Color____________________

Lips (color, brand, etc.)

Lip Liner ____________________

Lip Color ____________________

Gloss ____________________

Eyes (color, brand, etc.)

Brows ____________________

Lid Color 1 ____________________

Lid Color 2 ____________________

Lid Color 3 ____________________

Crease____________________

Eye Liner____________________

Mascara ____________________

Face (color, brand, etc.)

Concealer____________________

Foundation____________________

Contour____________________

Blush ____________________

Highlights ____________________

Powder____________________

Design/Client Name____________________ Date____________

Concealer	Foundation	Contour	Blush	Highlights	Powder	Eye Liner	Mascara
Brows	Lid Color 1	Lid Color 2	Lid Color 3	Crease	Lip Liner	Lip Color	Lip Gloss

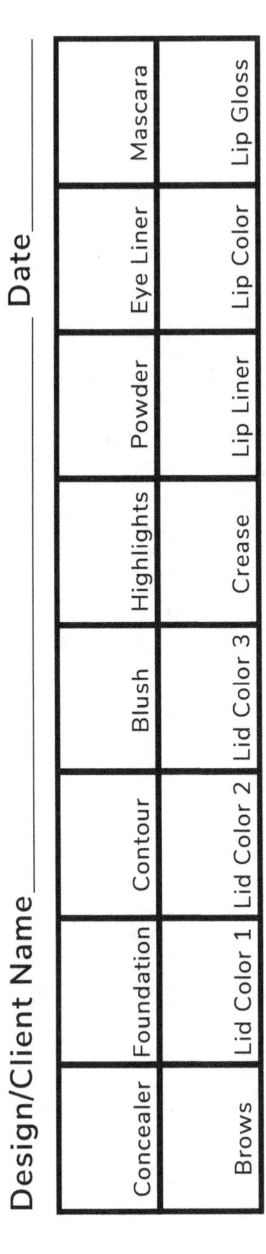

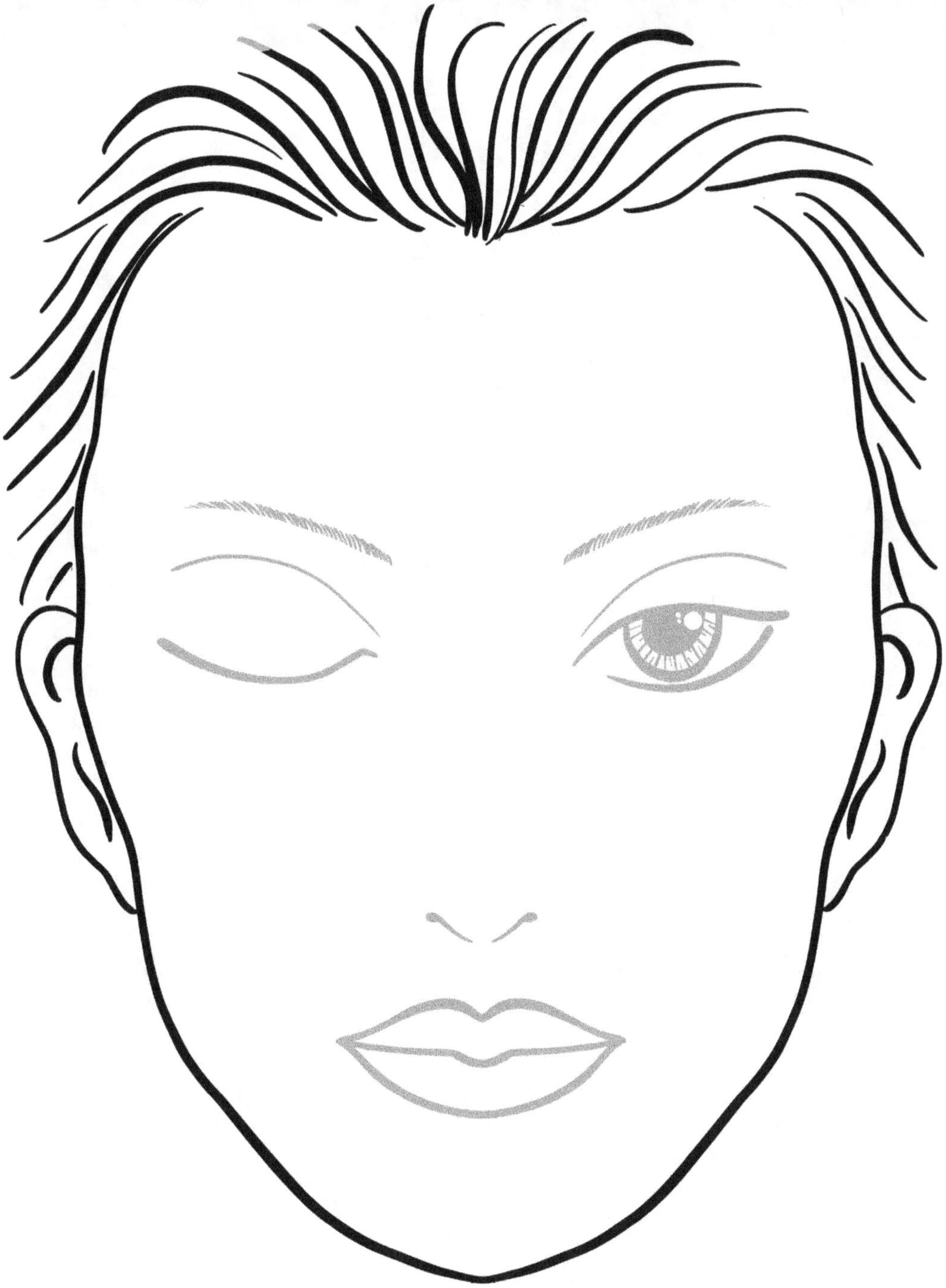

Details

Skin Tone____________________

Eye Color ____________________

Hair Color____________________

Lips (color, brand, etc.)

Lip Liner ____________________

Lip Color ____________________

Gloss ____________________

Eyes (color, brand, etc.)

Brows ____________________

Lid Color 1 ____________________

Lid Color 2 ____________________

Lid Color 3 ____________________

Crease____________________

Eye Liner____________________

Mascara ____________________

Face (color, brand, etc.)

Concealer____________________

Foundation____________________

Contour____________________

Blush ____________________

Highlights ____________________

Powder____________________

Design/Client Name____________ Date____________

Concealer	Brows
Foundation	Lid Color 1
Contour	Lid Color 2
Blush	Lid Color 3
Highlights	Crease
Powder	Lip Liner
Eye Liner	Lip Color
Mascara	Lip Gloss

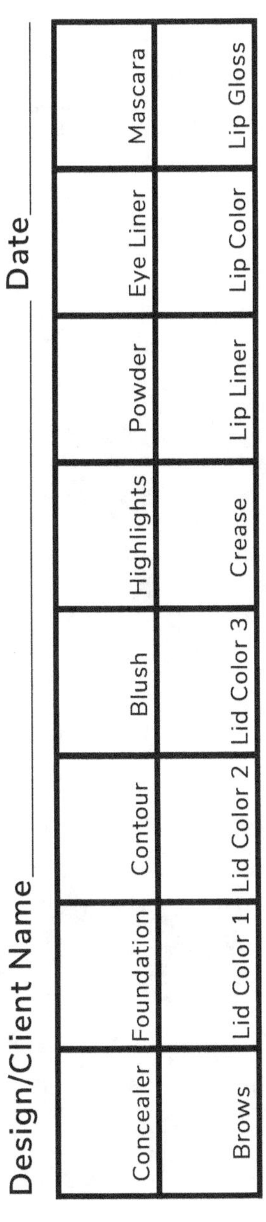

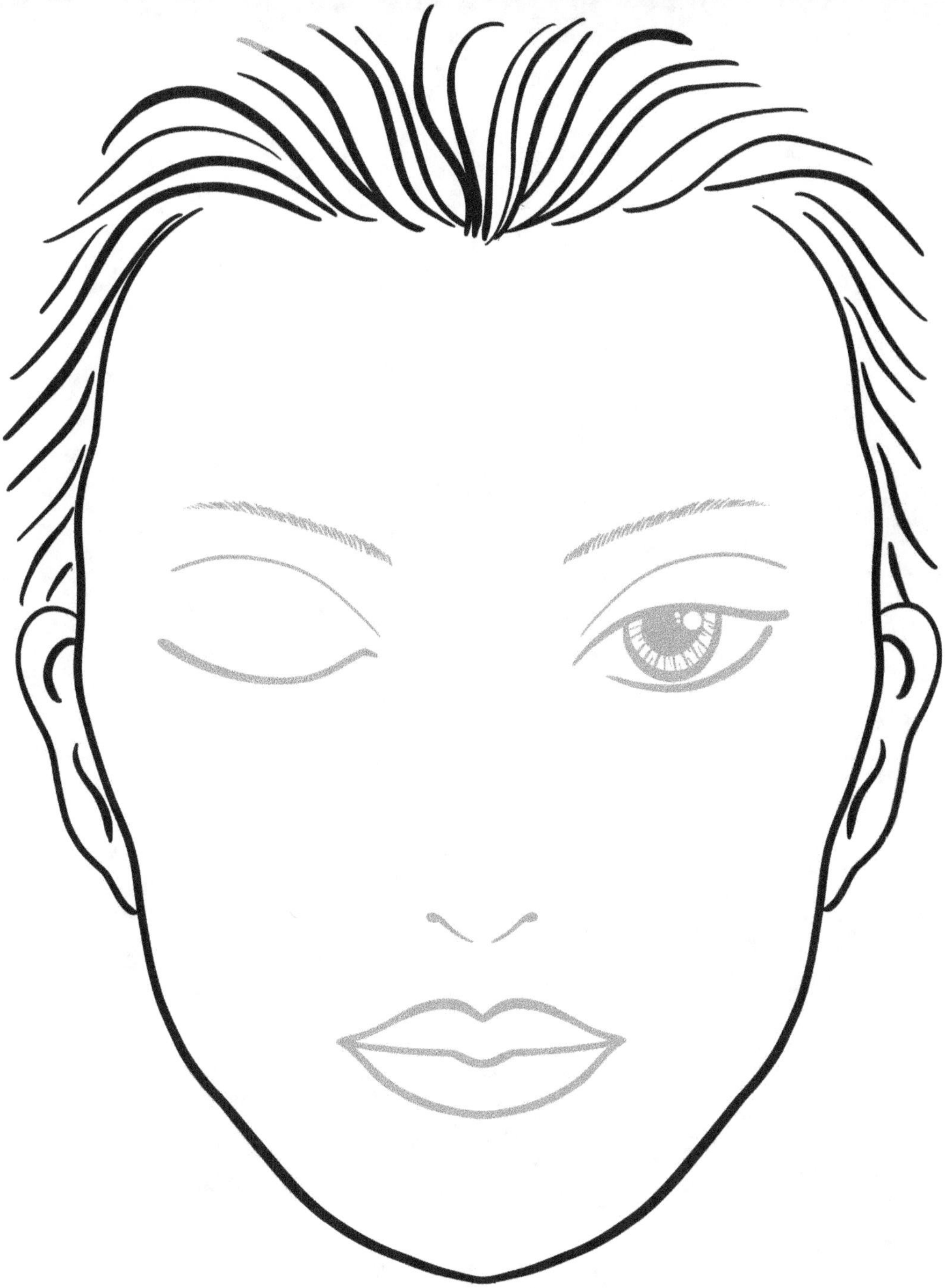

Details

Skin Tone____________________

Eye Color ____________________

Hair Color____________________

Lips (color, brand, etc.)

Lip Liner ____________________

Lip Color ____________________

Gloss ____________________

Eyes (color, brand, etc.)

Brows ____________________

Lid Color 1 ____________________

Lid Color 2 ____________________

Lid Color 3 ____________________

Crease____________________

Eye Liner____________________

Mascara ____________________

Face (color, brand, etc.)

Concealer____________________

Foundation____________________

Contour____________________

Blush ____________________

Highlights ____________________

Powder____________________

Design/Client Name ____________________ Date ____________

Concealer	Foundation	Contour	Blush	Highlights	Powder	Eye Liner	Mascara
Brows	Lid Color 1	Lid Color 2	Lid Color 3	Crease	Lip Liner	Lip Color	Lip Gloss

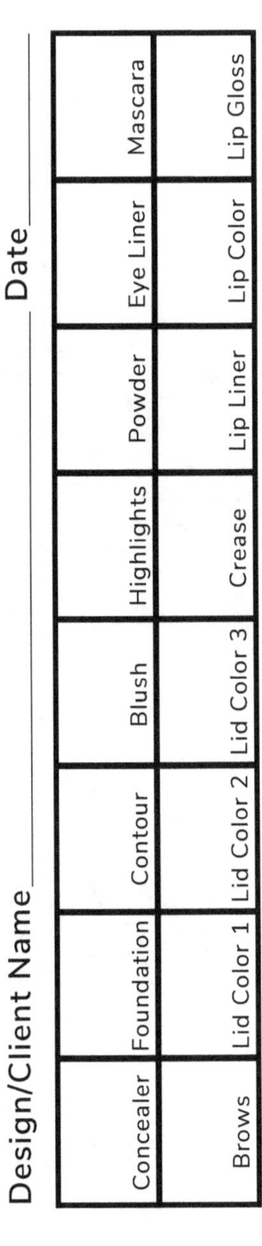

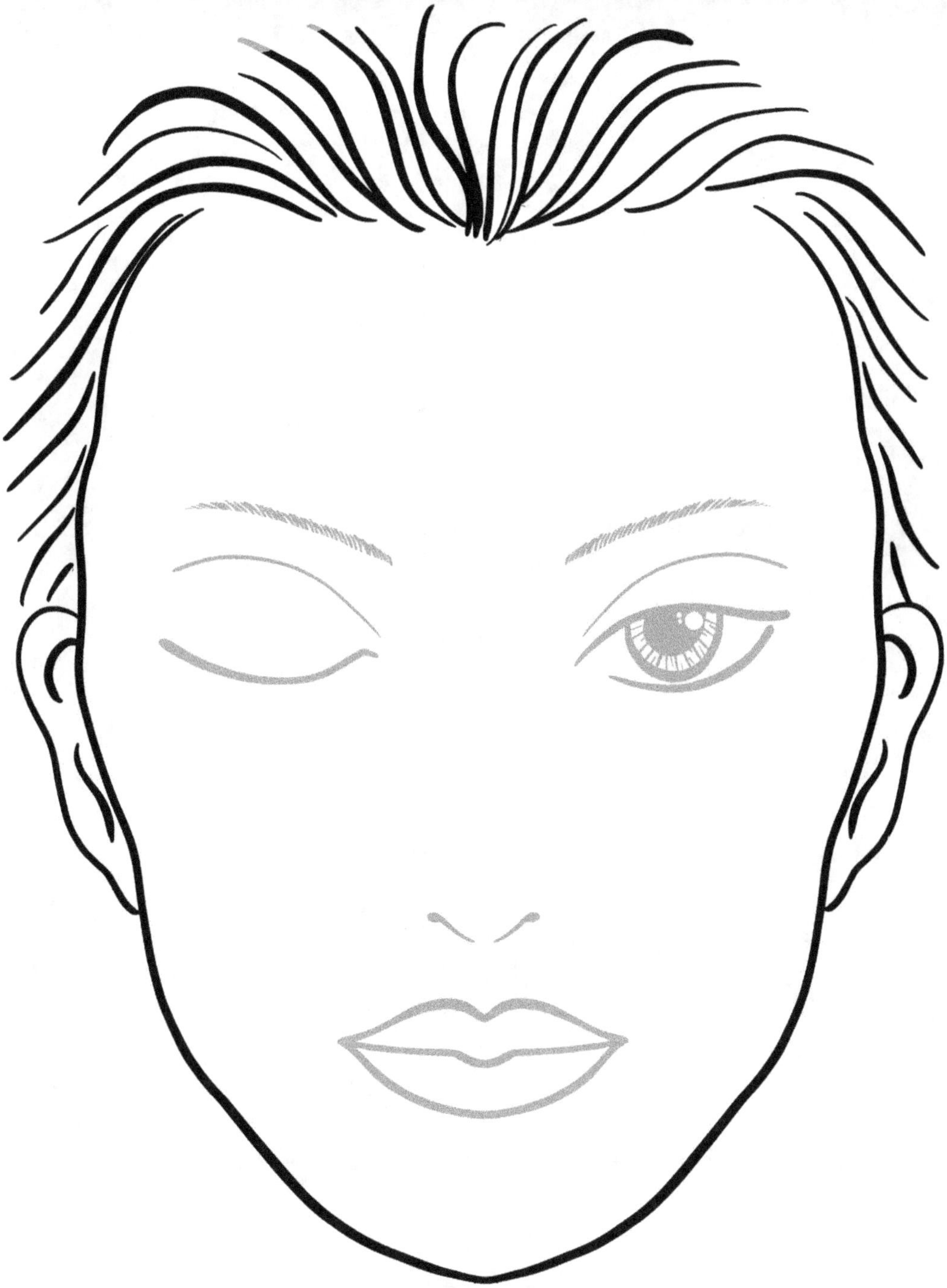

Details

Skin Tone ____________________

Eye Color ____________________

Hair Color ____________________

Lips (color, brand, etc.)

Lip Liner ____________________

Lip Color ____________________

Gloss ____________________

Eyes (color, brand, etc.)

Brows ____________________

Lid Color 1 ____________________

Lid Color 2 ____________________

Lid Color 3 ____________________

Crease ____________________

Eye Liner ____________________

Mascara ____________________

Face (color, brand, etc.)

Concealer ____________________

Foundation ____________________

Contour ____________________

Blush ____________________

Highlights ____________________

Powder ____________________

Design/Client Name________________ Date________

Concealer	Foundation	Contour	Blush	Highlights	Powder	Eye Liner	Mascara
Brows	Lid Color 1	Lid Color 2	Lid Color 3	Crease	Lip Liner	Lip Color	Lip Gloss

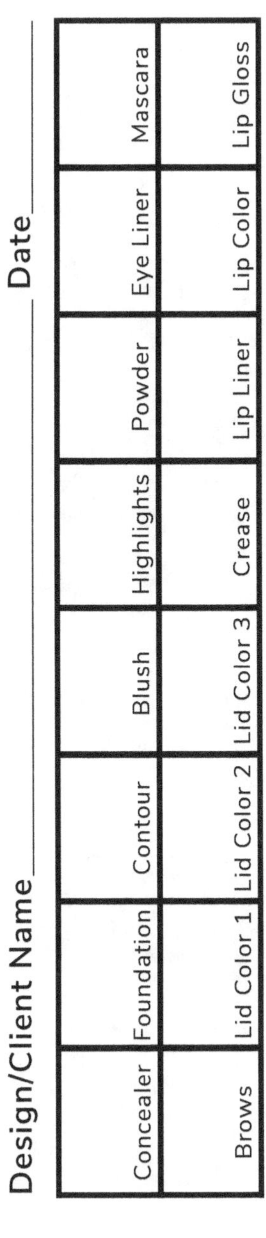

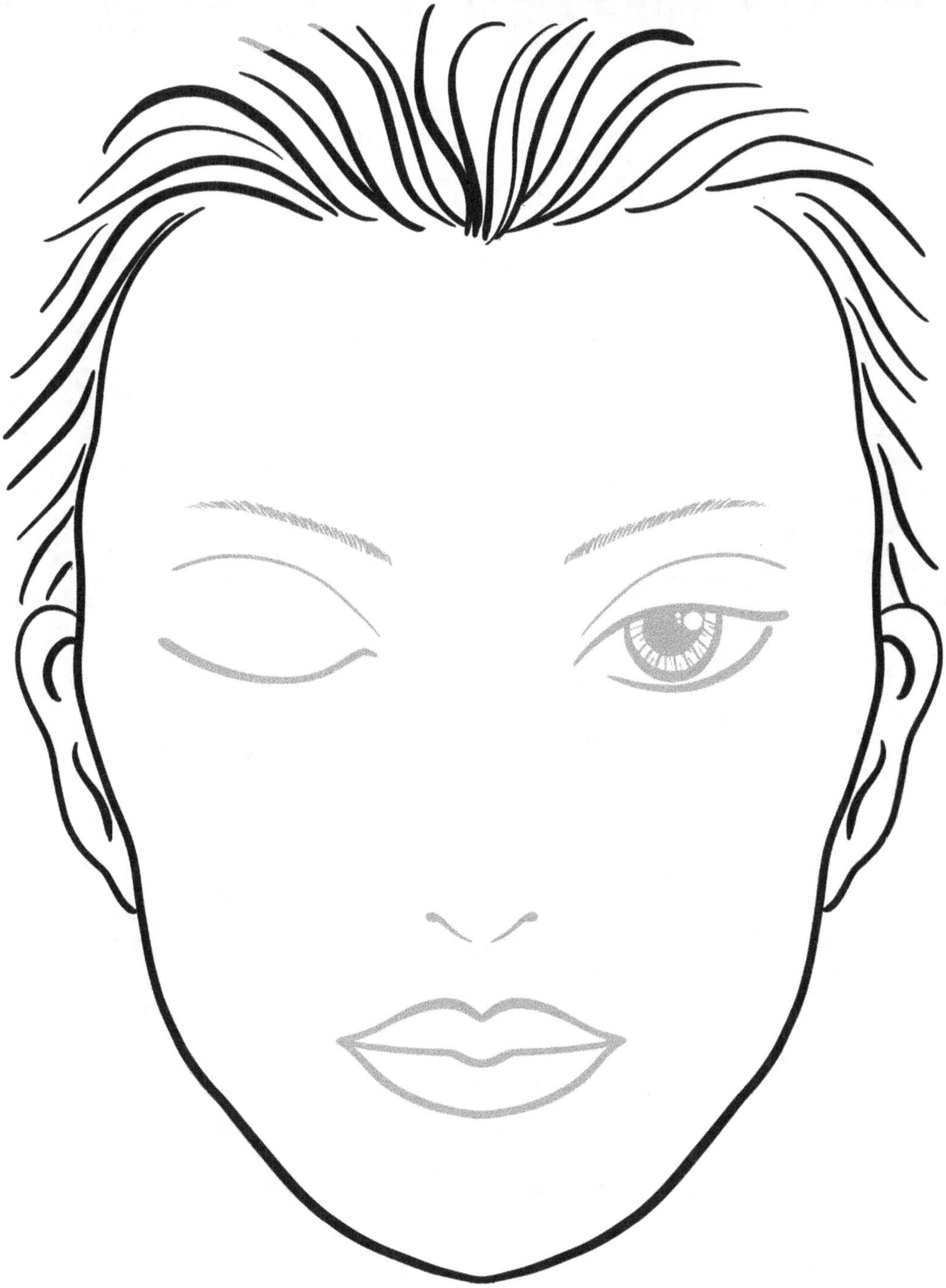

Details

Skin Tone____________________

Eye Color ____________________

Hair Color____________________

Lips (color, brand, etc.)

Lip Liner ____________________

Lip Color ____________________

Gloss ____________________

Eyes (color, brand, etc.)

Brows ____________________

Lid Color 1 ____________________

Lid Color 2 ____________________

Lid Color 3 ____________________

Crease____________________

Eye Liner____________________

Mascara ____________________

Face (color, brand, etc.)

Concealer____________________

Foundation____________________

Contour____________________

Blush ____________________

Highlights ____________________

Powder____________________

Design/Client Name ____________ Date ____________

Concealer	Foundation	Contour	Blush	Highlights	Powder	Eye Liner	Mascara
Brows	Lid Color 1	Lid Color 2	Lid Color 3	Crease	Lip Liner	Lip Color	Lip Gloss

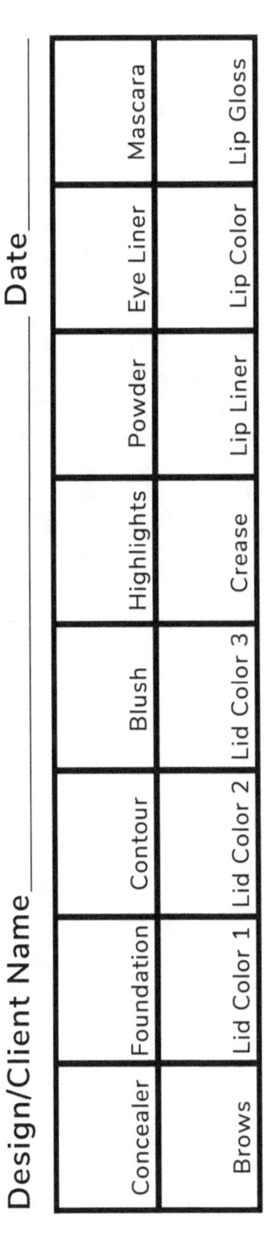

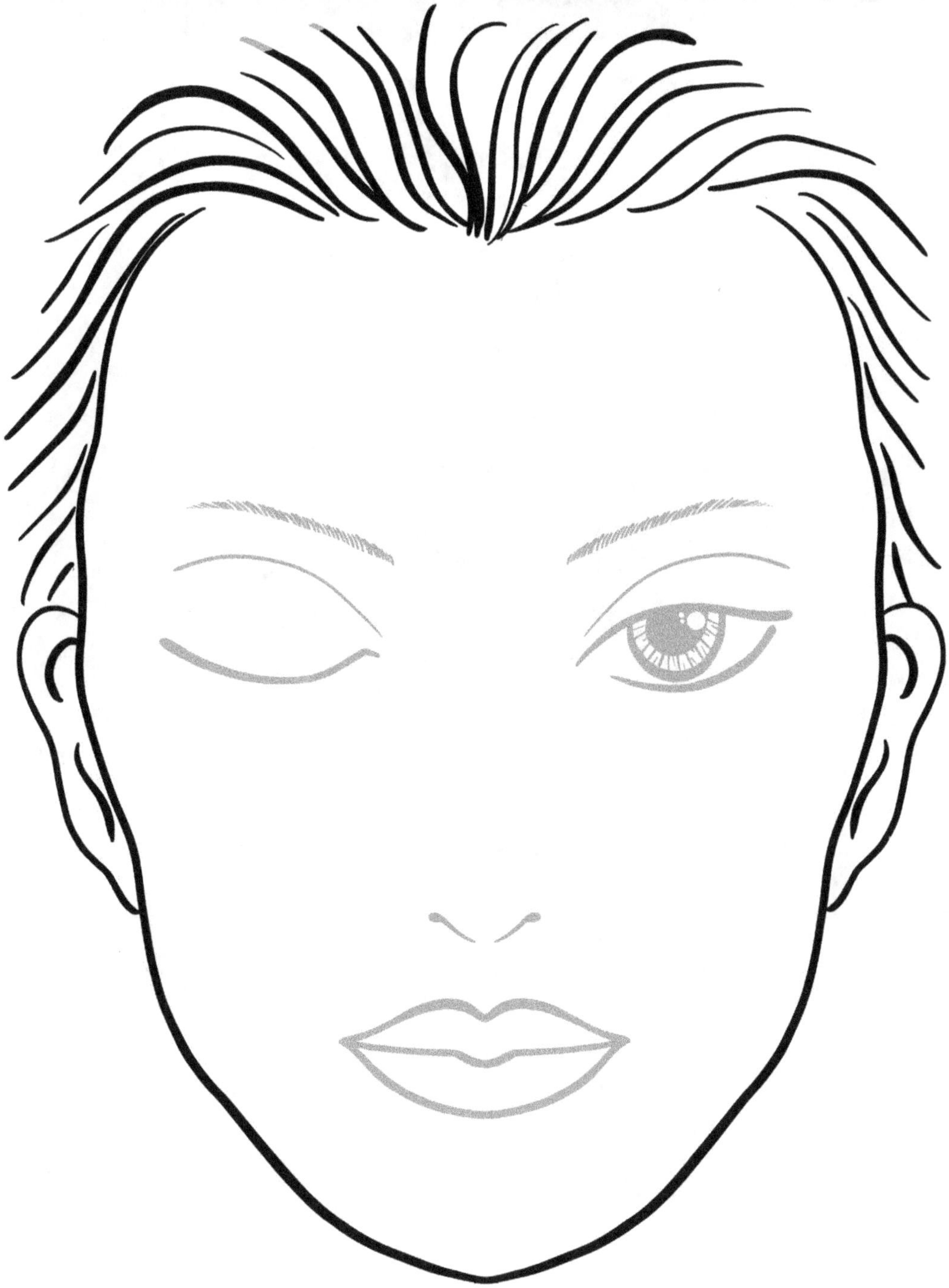

Details

Skin Tone ____________________

Eye Color ____________________

Hair Color ____________________

Lips (color, brand, etc.)

Lip Liner ____________________

Lip Color ____________________

Gloss ____________________

Eyes (color, brand, etc.)

Brows ____________________

Lid Color 1 ____________________

Lid Color 2 ____________________

Lid Color 3 ____________________

Crease ____________________

Eye Liner ____________________

Mascara ____________________

Face (color, brand, etc.)

Concealer ____________________

Foundation ____________________

Contour ____________________

Blush ____________________

Highlights ____________________

Powder ____________________

Design/Client Name________________ Date________________

Concealer	Foundation	Contour	Blush	Highlights	Powder	Eye Liner	Mascara
Brows	Lid Color 1	Lid Color 2	Lid Color 3	Crease	Lip Liner	Lip Color	Lip Gloss

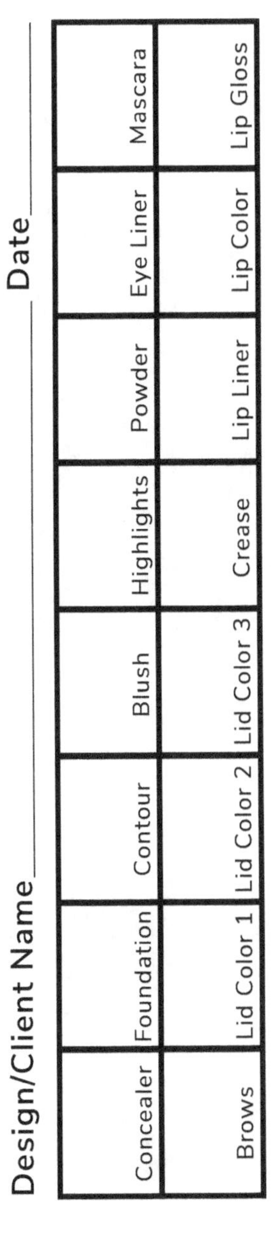

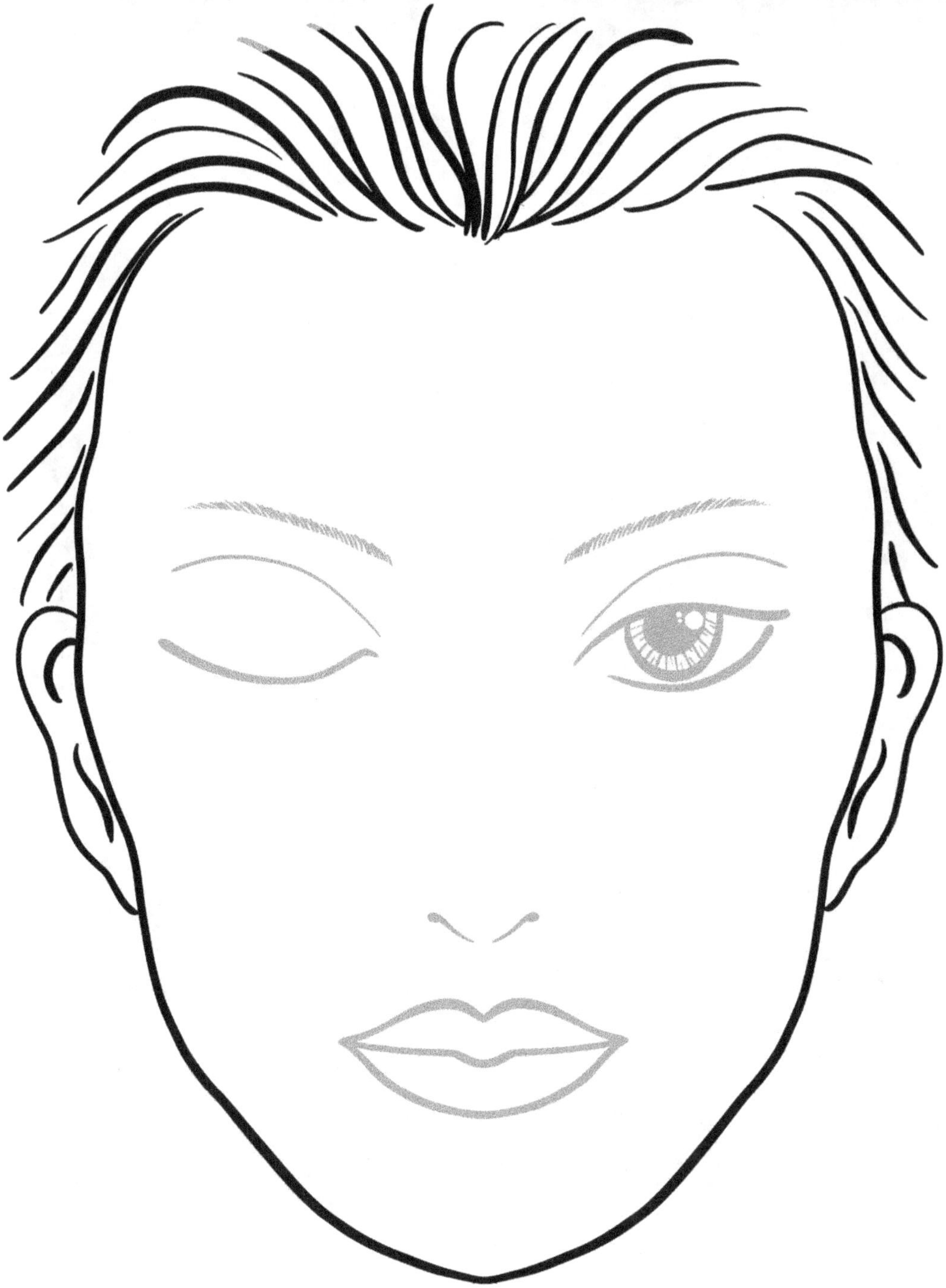

Details

Skin Tone____________________

Eye Color ____________________

Hair Color____________________

Lips (color, brand, etc.)

Lip Liner ____________________

Lip Color ____________________

Gloss ____________________

Eyes (color, brand, etc.)

Brows ____________________

Lid Color 1 ____________________

Lid Color 2 ____________________

Lid Color 3 ____________________

Crease____________________

Eye Liner____________________

Mascara ____________________

Face (color, brand, etc.)

Concealer____________________

Foundation____________________

Contour____________________

Blush ____________________

Highlights ____________________

Powder____________________

Design/Client Name____________________ Date____________

Concealer	Foundation	Contour	Blush	Highlights	Powder	Eye Liner	Mascara
Brows	Lid Color 1	Lid Color 2	Lid Color 3	Crease	Lip Liner	Lip Color	Lip Gloss

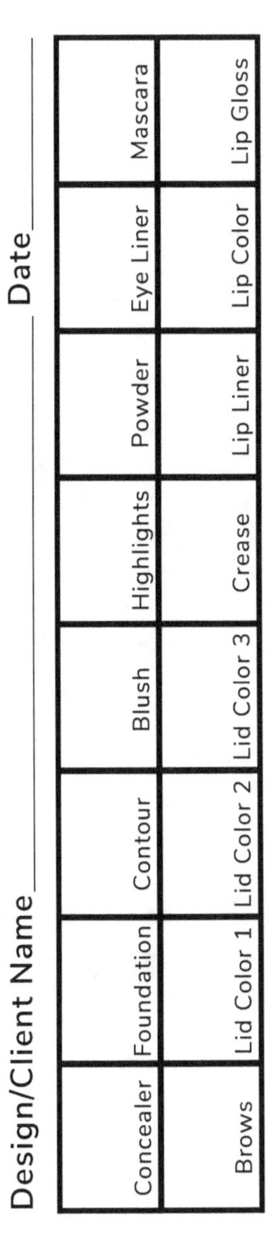

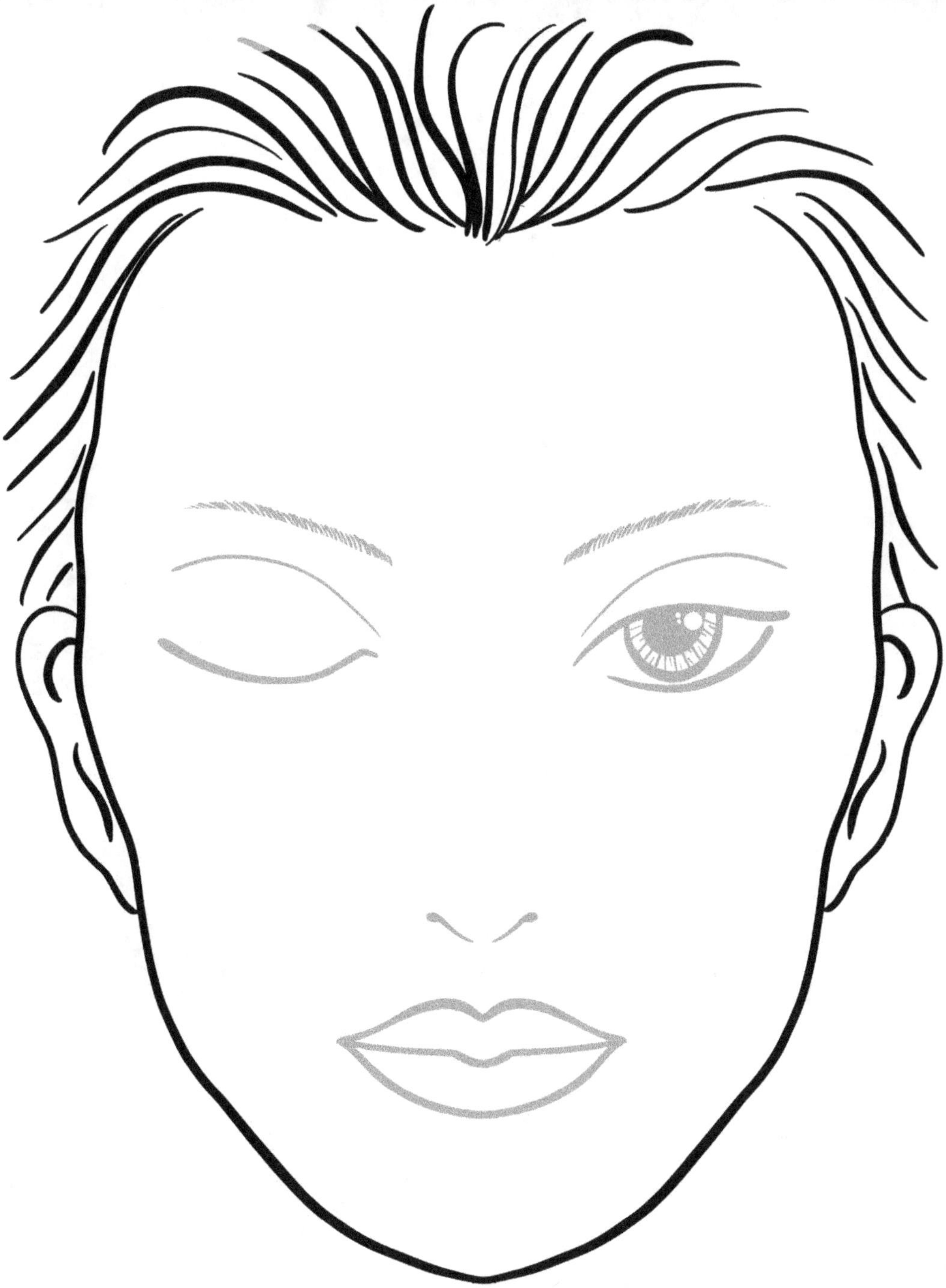

Details

Skin Tone____________________

Eye Color ____________________

Hair Color____________________

Lips (color, brand, etc.)

Lip Liner ____________________

Lip Color ____________________

Gloss ____________________

Eyes (color, brand, etc.)

Brows ____________________

Lid Color 1 ____________________

Lid Color 2 ____________________

Lid Color 3 ____________________

Crease____________________

Eye Liner____________________

Mascara ____________________

Face (color, brand, etc.)

Concealer____________________

Foundation____________________

Contour____________________

Blush ____________________

Highlights ____________________

Powder____________________

Design/Client Name______________ Date______________

Concealer	Foundation	Contour	Blush	Highlights	Powder	Eye Liner	Mascara
Brows	Lid Color 1	Lid Color 2	Lid Color 3	Crease	Lip Liner	Lip Color	Lip Gloss

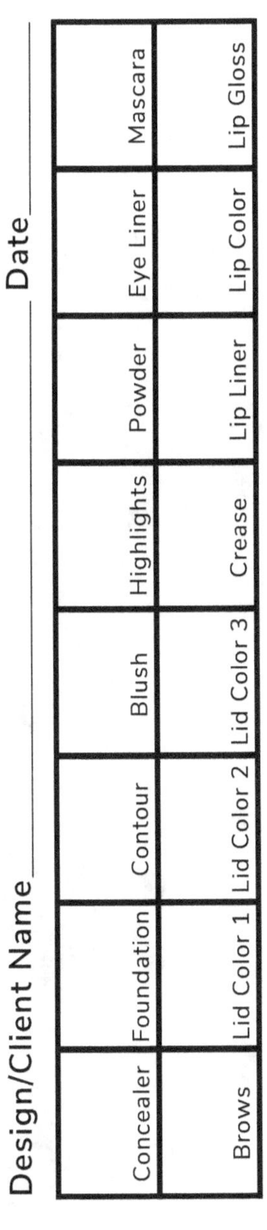

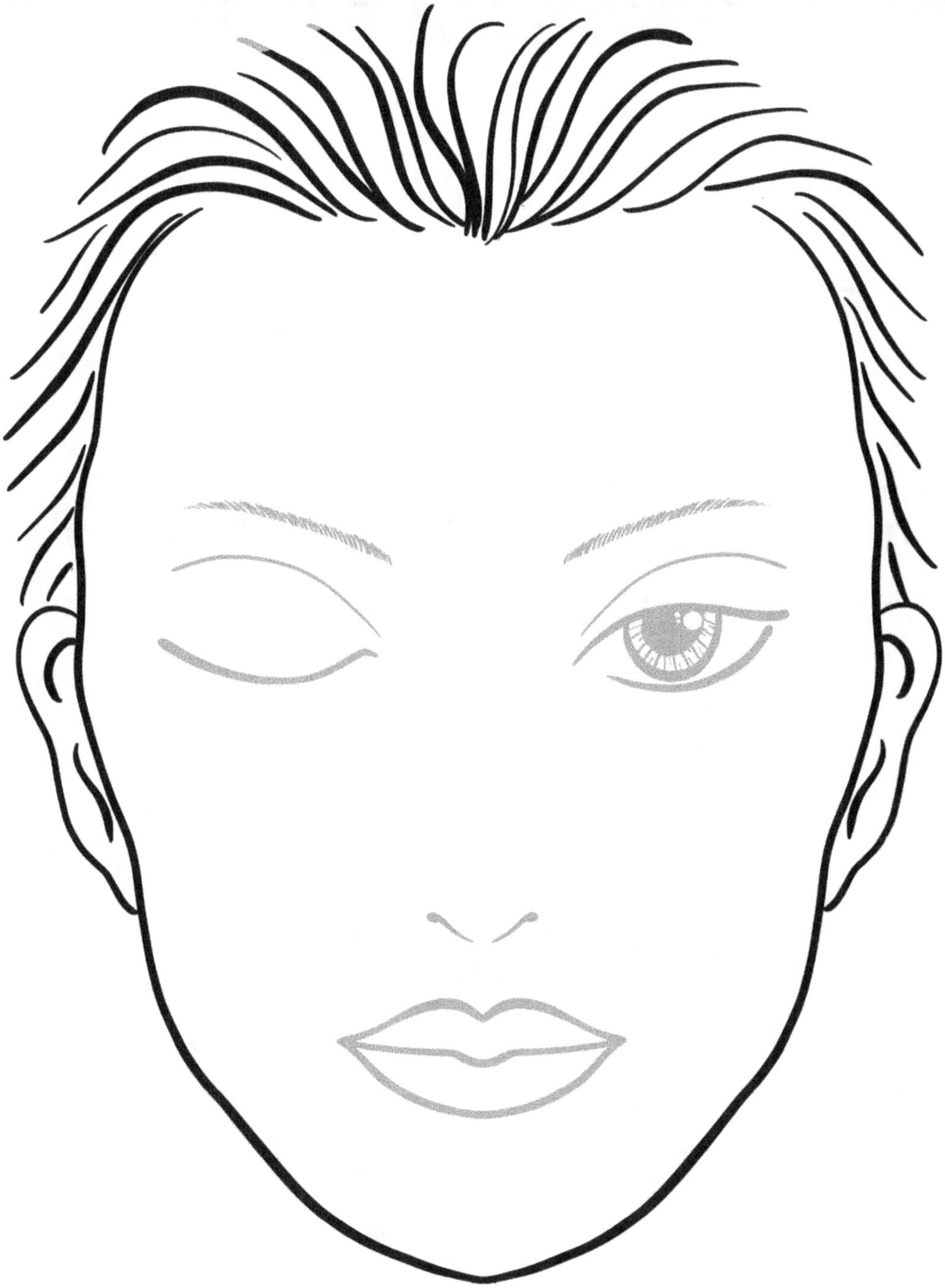

Details

Skin Tone____________________

Eye Color ____________________

Hair Color____________________

Lips (color, brand, etc.)

Lip Liner ____________________

Lip Color ____________________

Gloss ____________________

Eyes (color, brand, etc.)

Brows ____________________

Lid Color 1 ____________________

Lid Color 2 ____________________

Lid Color 3 ____________________

Crease____________________

Eye Liner____________________

Mascara ____________________

Face (color, brand, etc.)

Concealer____________________

Foundation____________________

Contour____________________

Blush ____________________

Highlights ____________________

Powder____________________

Design/Client Name____________________ Date____________

Concealer	Foundation	Contour	Blush	Highlights	Powder	Eye Liner	Mascara
Brows	Lid Color 1	Lid Color 2	Lid Color 3	Crease	Lip Liner	Lip Color	Lip Gloss

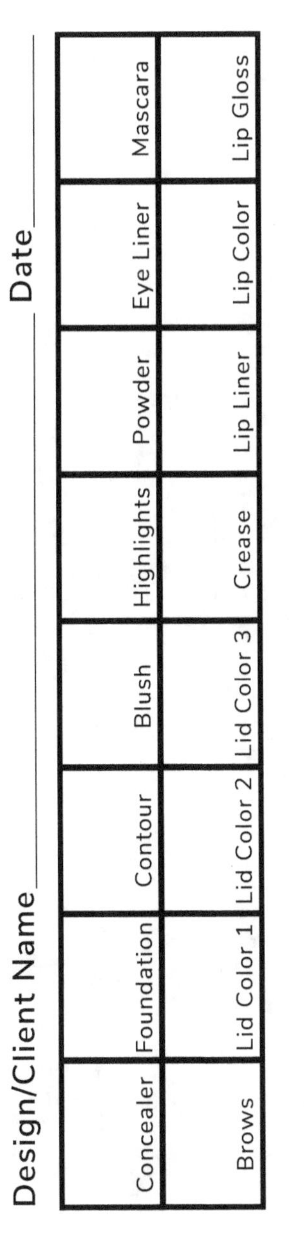

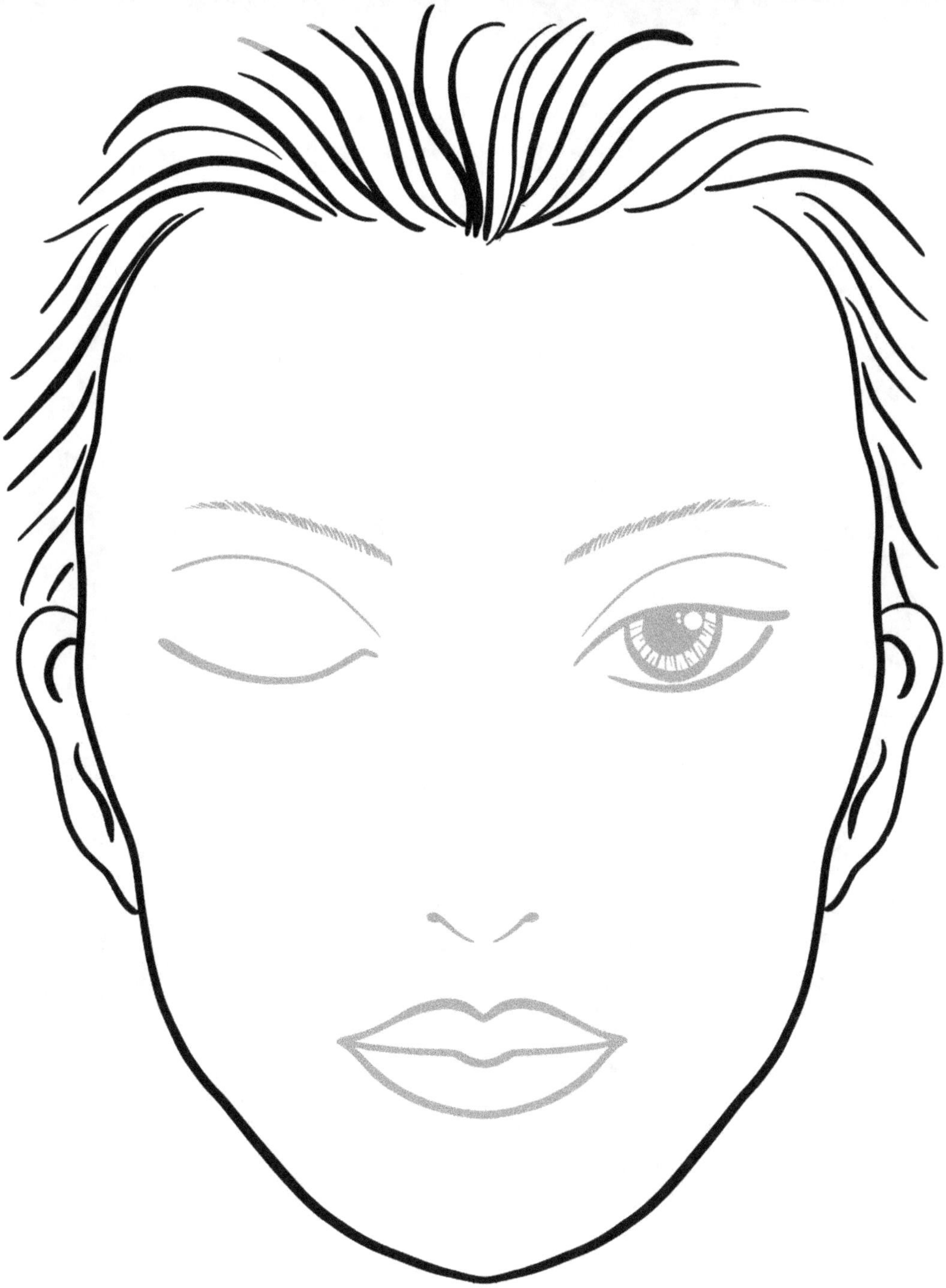

Details

Skin Tone____________________

Eye Color ____________________

Hair Color____________________

Lips (color, brand, etc.)

Lip Liner ____________________

Lip Color ____________________

Gloss ____________________

Eyes (color, brand, etc.)

Brows ____________________

Lid Color 1 ____________________

Lid Color 2 ____________________

Lid Color 3 ____________________

Crease____________________

Eye Liner____________________

Mascara____________________

Face (color, brand, etc.)

Concealer____________________

Foundation____________________

Contour____________________

Blush ____________________

Highlights ____________________

Powder____________________

Design/Client Name________________ Date________________

Concealer	Brows
Foundation	Lid Color 1
Contour	Lid Color 2
Blush	Lid Color 3
Highlights	Crease
Powder	Lip Liner
Eye Liner	Lip Color
Mascara	Lip Gloss

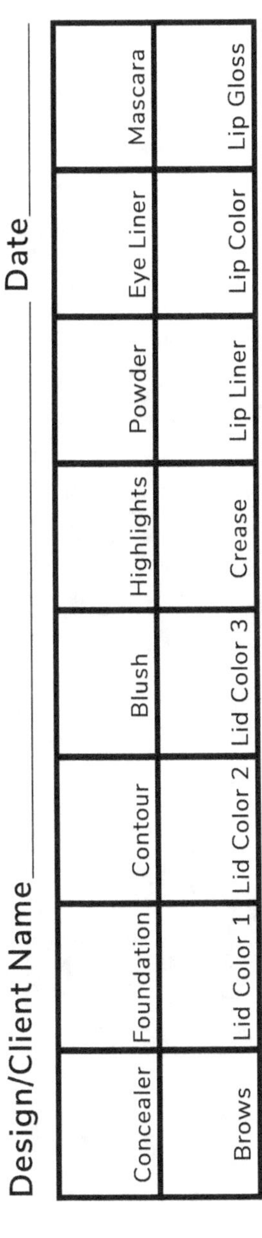

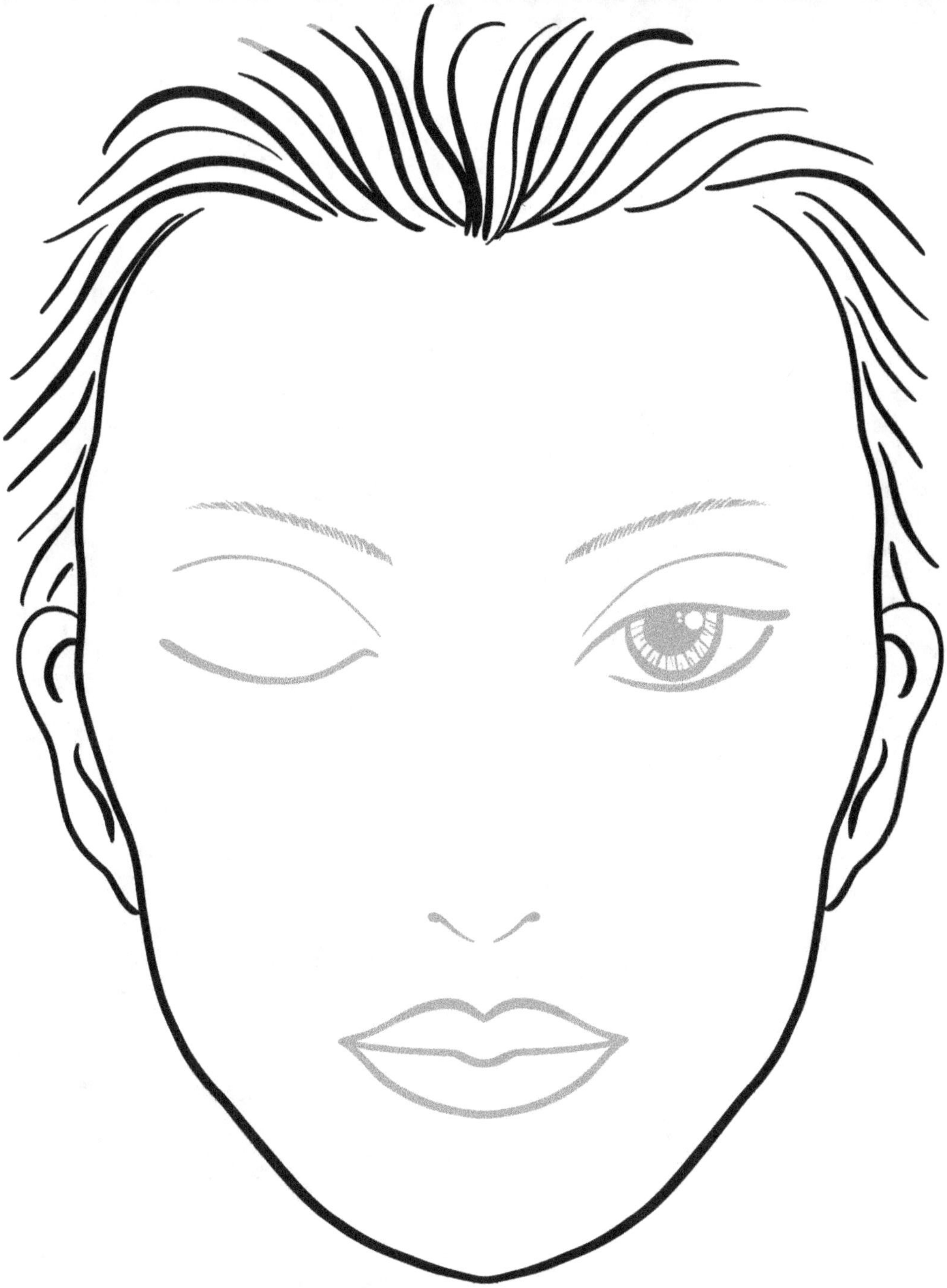

Details

Skin Tone________________

Eye Color ________________

Hair Color________________

Lips (color, brand, etc.)

Lip Liner ________________

Lip Color ________________

Gloss ________________

Eyes (color, brand, etc.)

Brows ________________

Lid Color 1 ________________

Lid Color 2 ________________

Lid Color 3 ________________

Crease________________

Eye Liner________________

Mascara ________________

Face (color, brand, etc.)

Concealer________________

Foundation________________

Contour________________

Blush ________________

Highlights ________________

Powder________________

Design/Client Name ____________ Date ____________

Concealer	Foundation	Contour	Blush	Highlights	Powder	Eye Liner	Mascara
Brows	Lid Color 1	Lid Color 2	Lid Color 3	Crease	Lip Liner	Lip Color	Lip Gloss

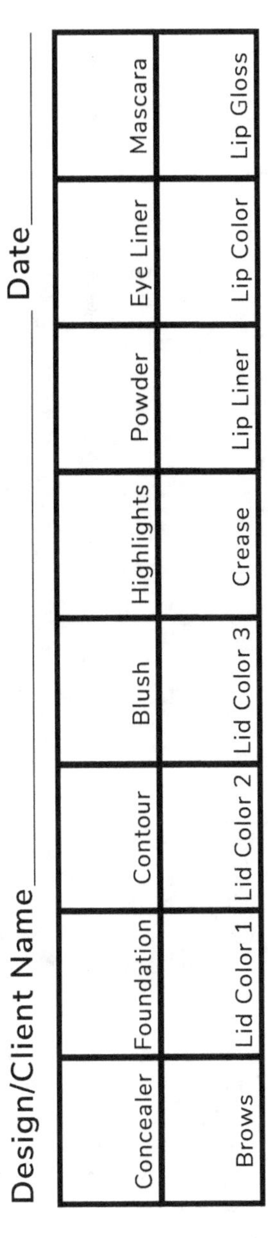

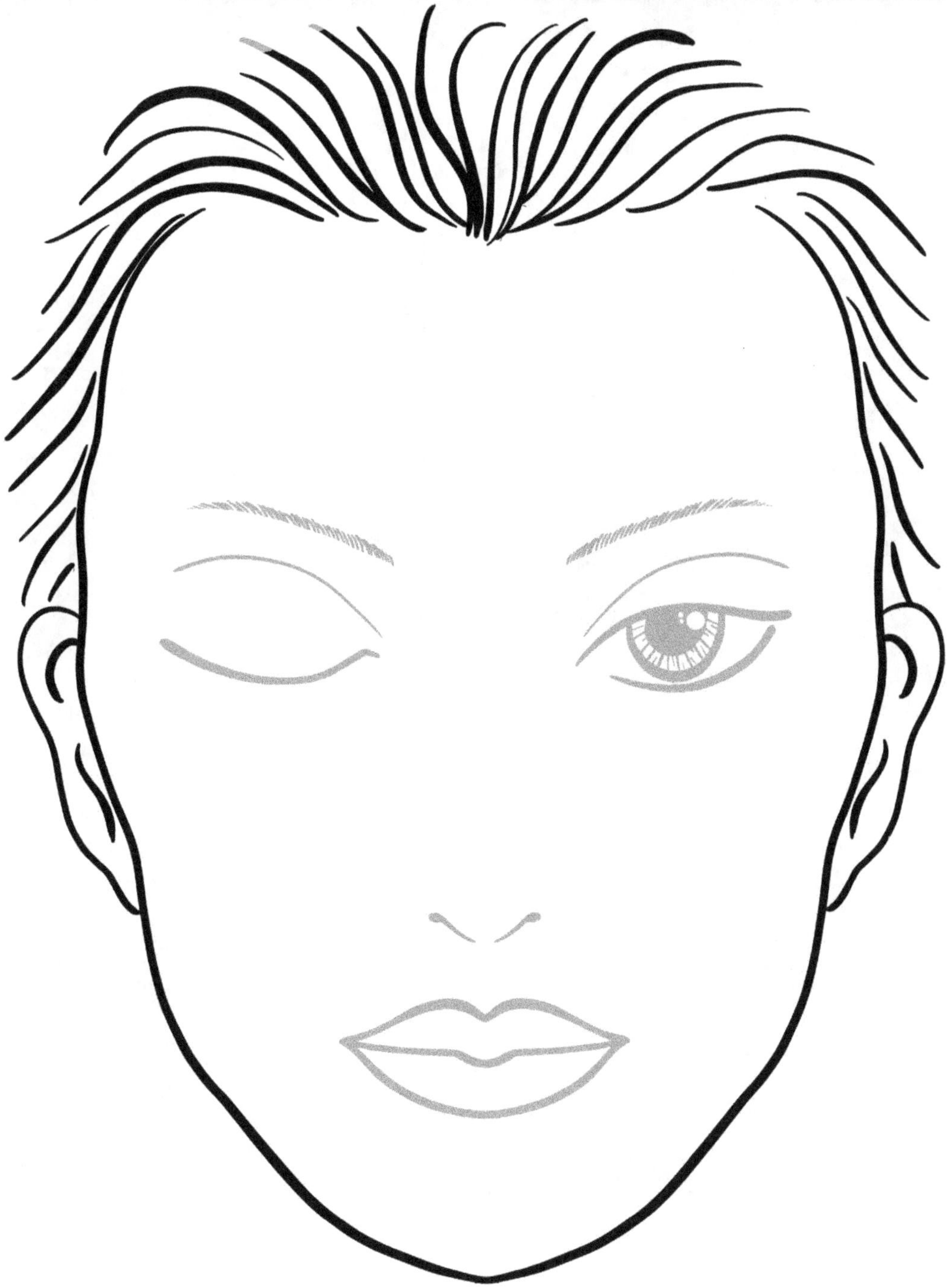

Details

Skin Tone ____________

Eye Color ____________

Hair Color ____________

Lips (color, brand, etc.)

Lip Liner ____________

Lip Color ____________

Gloss ____________

Eyes (color, brand, etc.)

Brows ____________

Lid Color 1 ____________

Lid Color 2 ____________

Lid Color 3 ____________

Crease ____________

Eye Liner ____________

Mascara ____________

Face (color, brand, etc.)

Concealer ____________

Foundation ____________

Contour ____________

Blush ____________

Highlights ____________

Powder ____________

Design/Client Name________________ Date________________

Concealer	Foundation	Contour	Blush	Highlights	Powder	Eye Liner	Mascara
Brows	Lid Color 1	Lid Color 2	Lid Color 3	Crease	Lip Liner	Lip Color	Lip Gloss

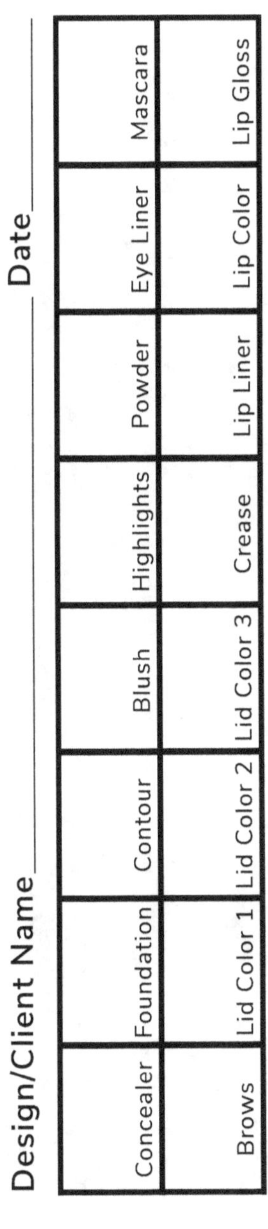

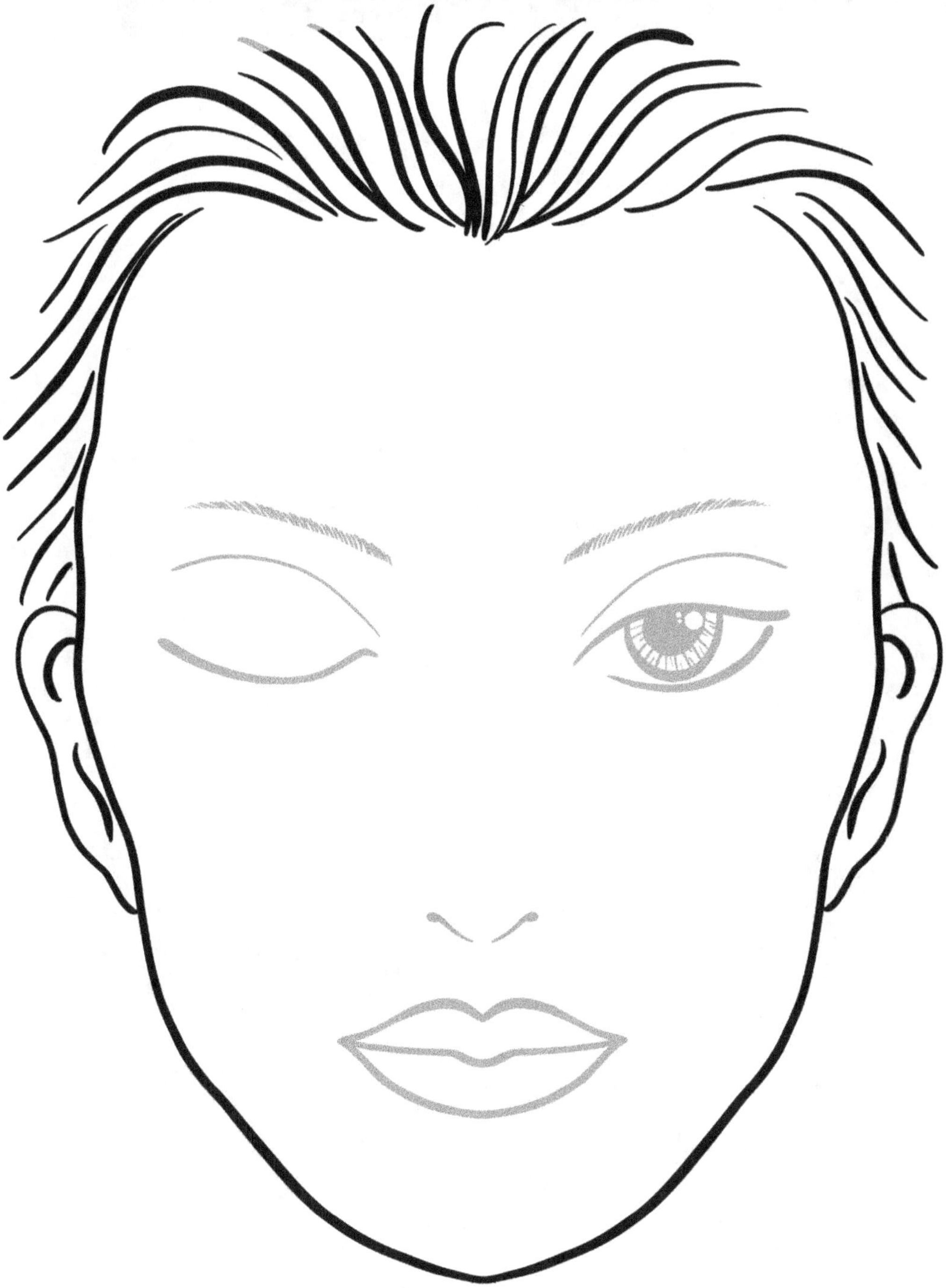

Details

Skin Tone____________________

Eye Color ____________________

Hair Color____________________

Lips (color, brand, etc.)

Lip Liner ____________________

Lip Color ____________________

Gloss ____________________

Eyes (color, brand, etc.)

Brows ____________________

Lid Color 1 ____________________

Lid Color 2 ____________________

Lid Color 3 ____________________

Crease____________________

Eye Liner____________________

Mascara ____________________

Face (color, brand, etc.)

Concealer____________________

Foundation____________________

Contour____________________

Blush ____________________

Highlights ____________________

Powder____________________

Design/Client Name ____________________ Date ____________

Concealer	Foundation	Contour	Blush	Highlights	Powder	Eye Liner	Mascara
Brows	Lid Color 1	Lid Color 2	Lid Color 3	Crease	Lip Liner	Lip Color	Lip Gloss

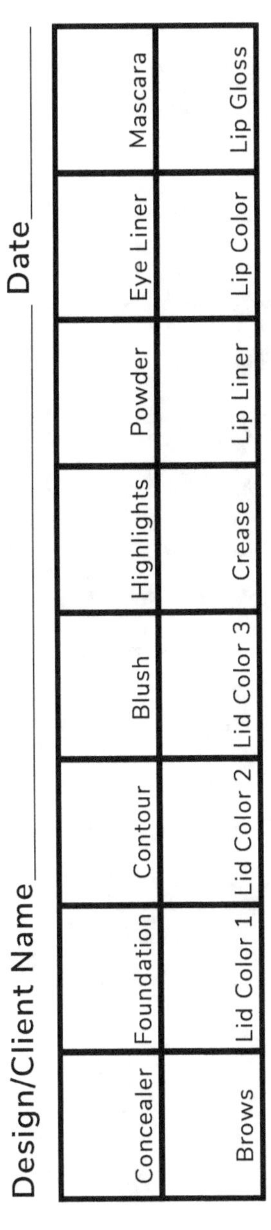

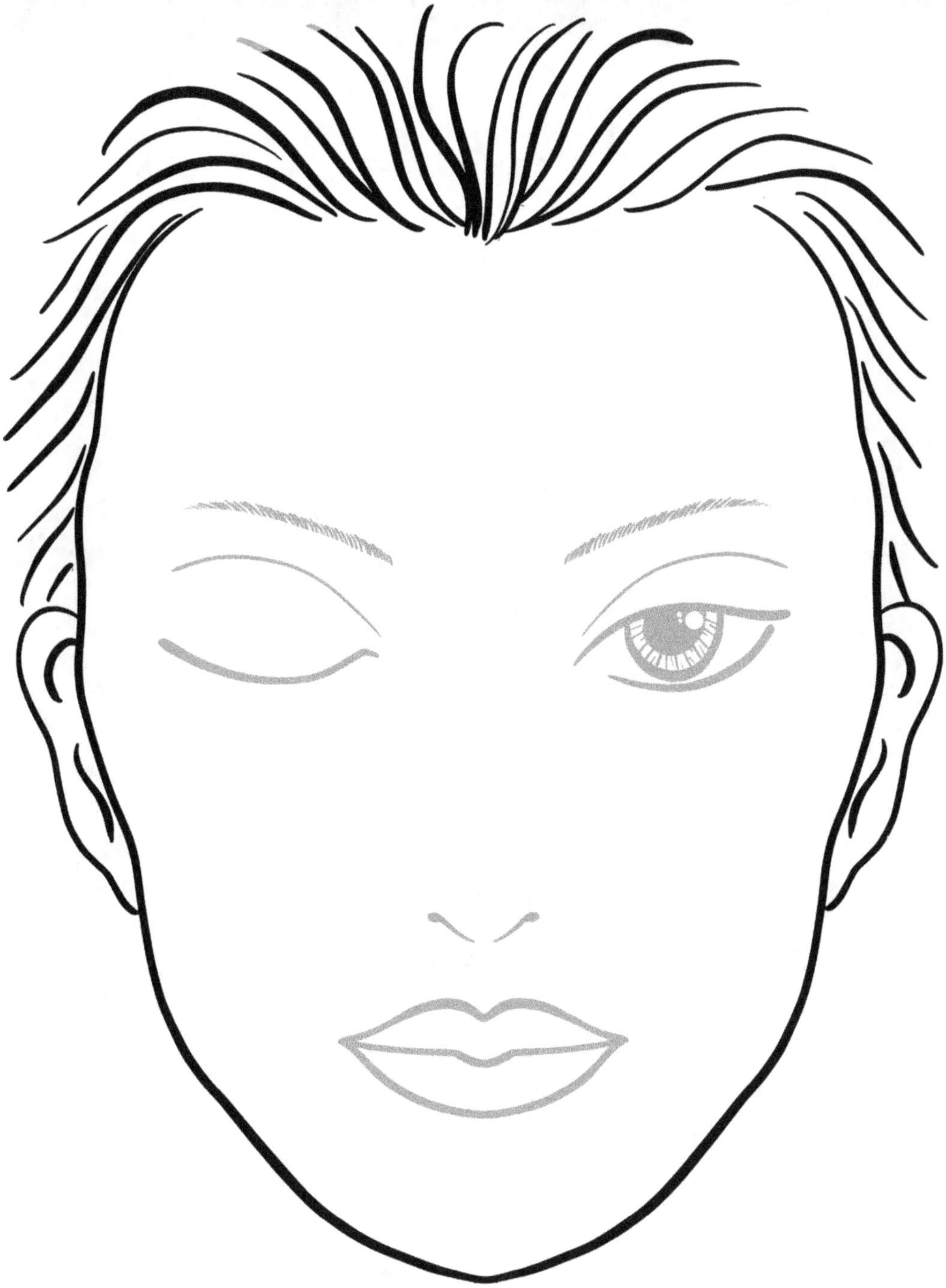

Details

Skin Tone ____________________

Eye Color ____________________

Hair Color ____________________

Lips (color, brand, etc.)

Lip Liner ____________________

Lip Color ____________________

Gloss ____________________

Eyes (color, brand, etc.)

Brows ____________________

Lid Color 1 ____________________

Lid Color 2 ____________________

Lid Color 3 ____________________

Crease ____________________

Eye Liner ____________________

Mascara ____________________

Face (color, brand, etc.)

Concealer ____________________

Foundation ____________________

Contour ____________________

Blush ____________________

Highlights ____________________

Powder ____________________

Design/Client Name________________ Date________________

Concealer	Foundation	Contour	Blush	Highlights	Powder	Eye Liner	Mascara
Brows	Lid Color 1	Lid Color 2	Lid Color 3	Crease	Lip Liner	Lip Color	Lip Gloss

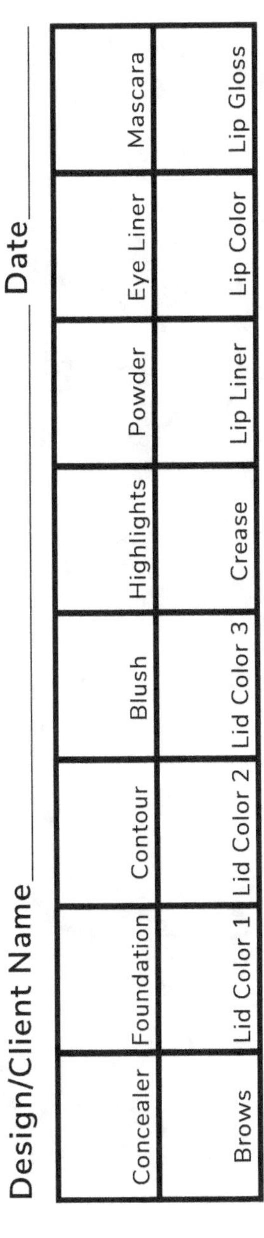

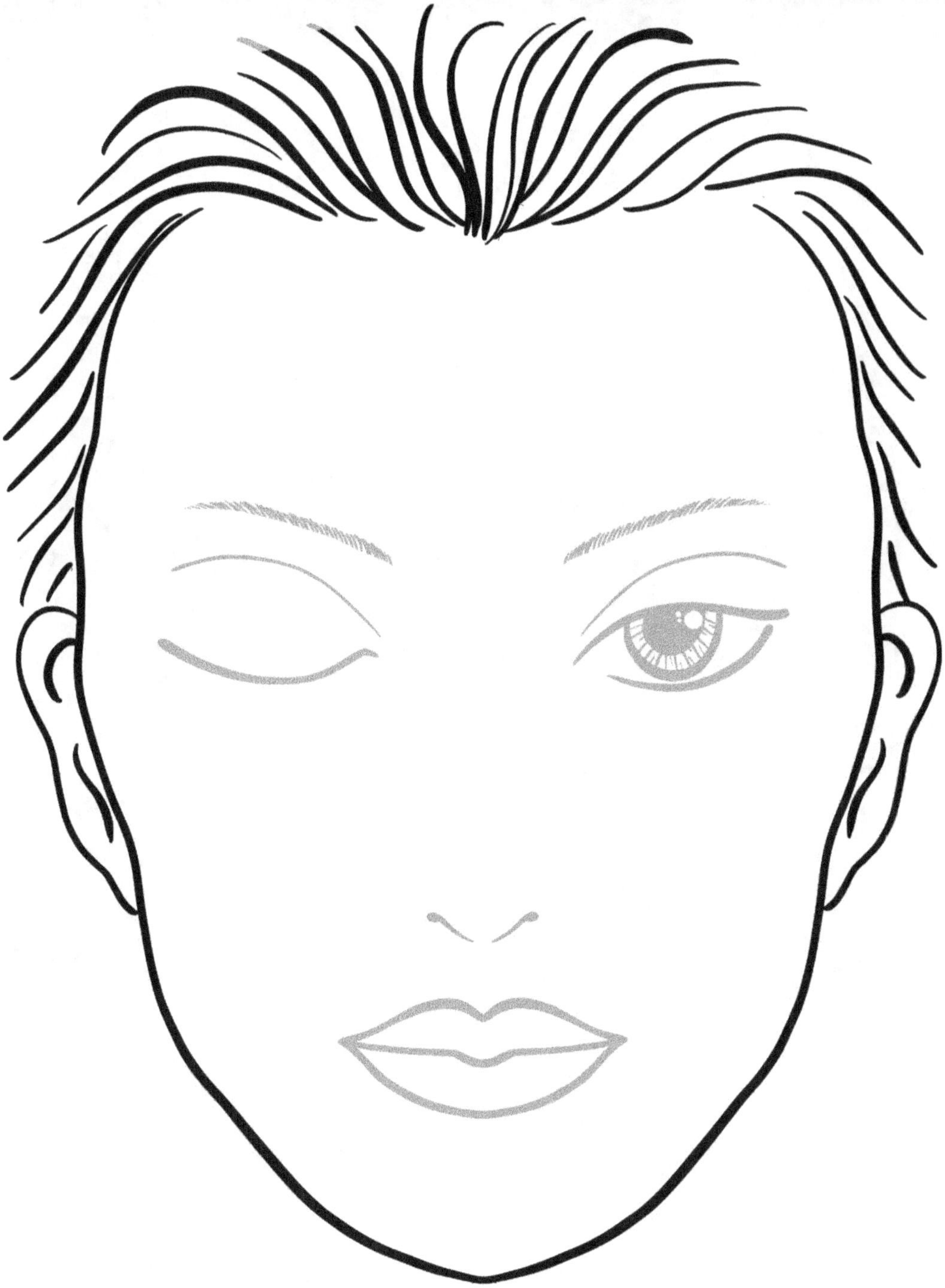

Details

Skin Tone____________________

Eye Color ____________________

Hair Color____________________

Lips (color, brand, etc.)

Lip Liner ____________________

Lip Color ____________________

Gloss ____________________

Eyes (color, brand, etc.)

Brows ____________________

Lid Color 1 ____________________

Lid Color 2 ____________________

Lid Color 3 ____________________

Crease ____________________

Eye Liner____________________

Mascara ____________________

Face (color, brand, etc.)

Concealer____________________

Foundation____________________

Contour____________________

Blush ____________________

Highlights ____________________

Powder____________________

Design/Client Name________________ Date________________

Concealer	Foundation	Contour	Blush	Highlights	Powder	Eye Liner	Mascara
Brows	Lid Color 1	Lid Color 2	Lid Color 3	Crease	Lip Liner	Lip Color	Lip Gloss

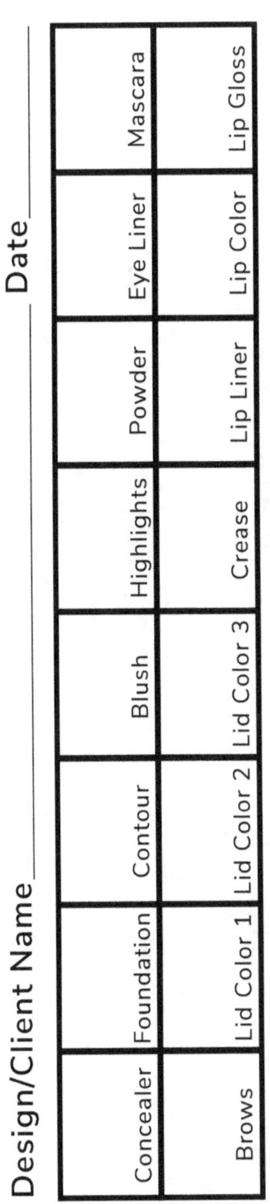

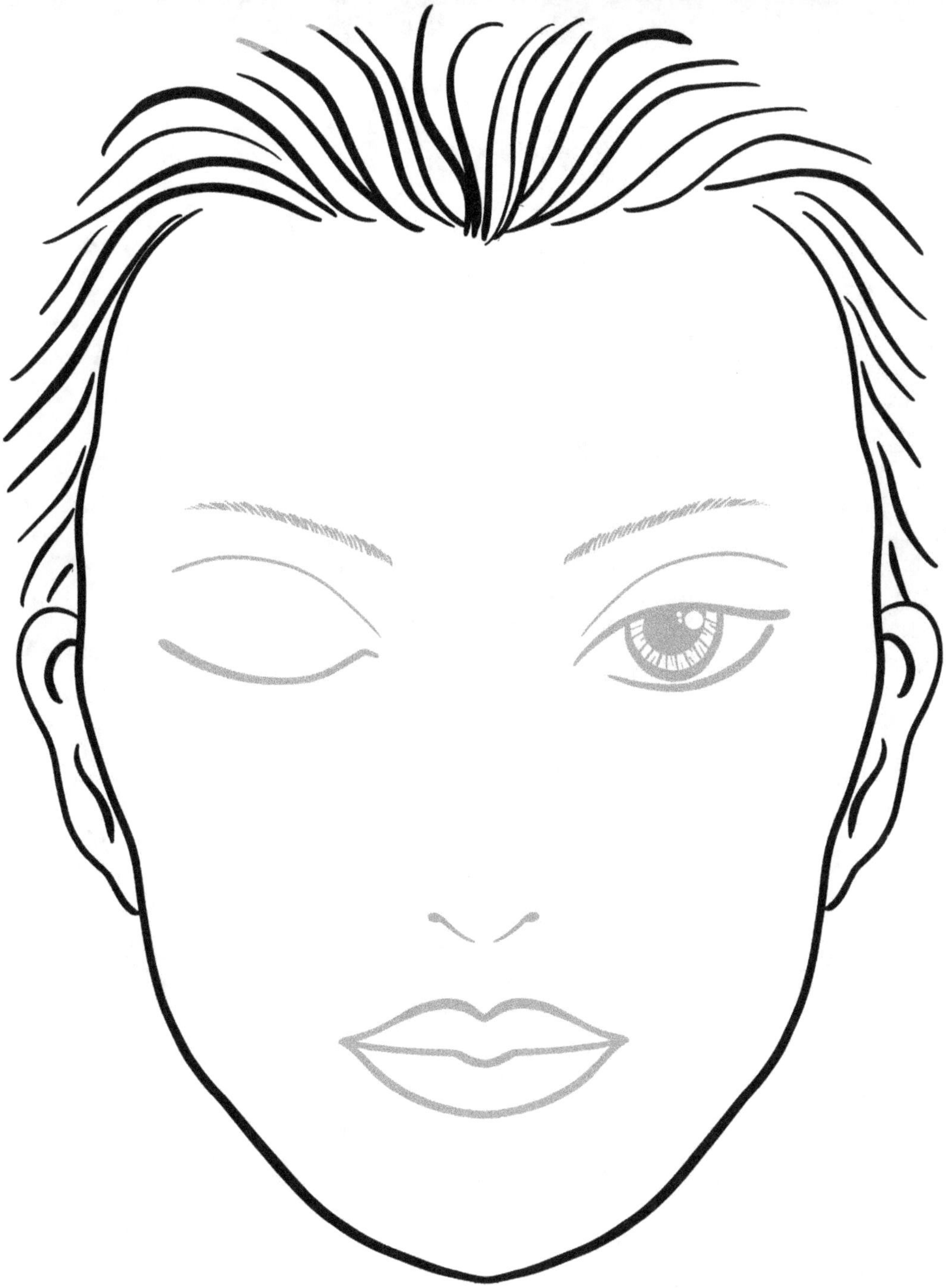

Details

Skin Tone________________________

Eye Color ________________________

Hair Color________________________

Lips (color, brand, etc.)

Lip Liner ________________________

Lip Color ________________________

Gloss ________________________

Eyes (color, brand, etc.)

Brows ________________________

Lid Color 1 ________________________

Lid Color 2 ________________________

Lid Color 3 ________________________

Crease________________________

Eye Liner________________________

Mascara ________________________

Face (color, brand, etc.)

Concealer________________________

Foundation________________________

Contour________________________

Blush ________________________

Highlights ________________________

Powder________________________

Design/Client Name____________ Date____________

Concealer	Foundation	Contour	Blush	Highlights	Powder	Eye Liner	Mascara
Brows	Lid Color 1	Lid Color 2	Lid Color 3	Crease	Lip Liner	Lip Color	Lip Gloss

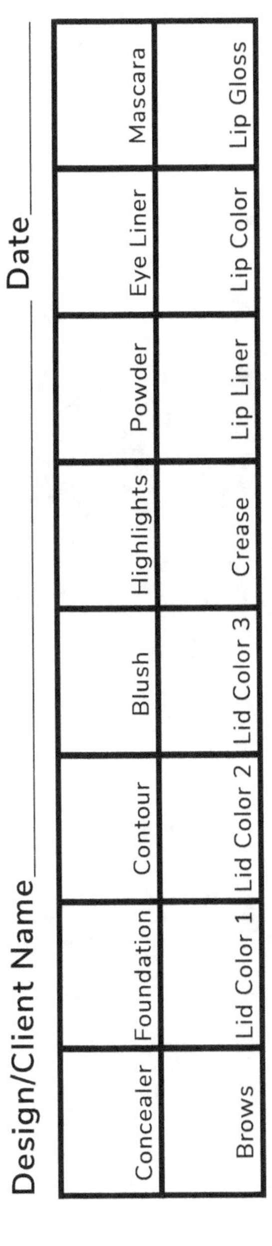

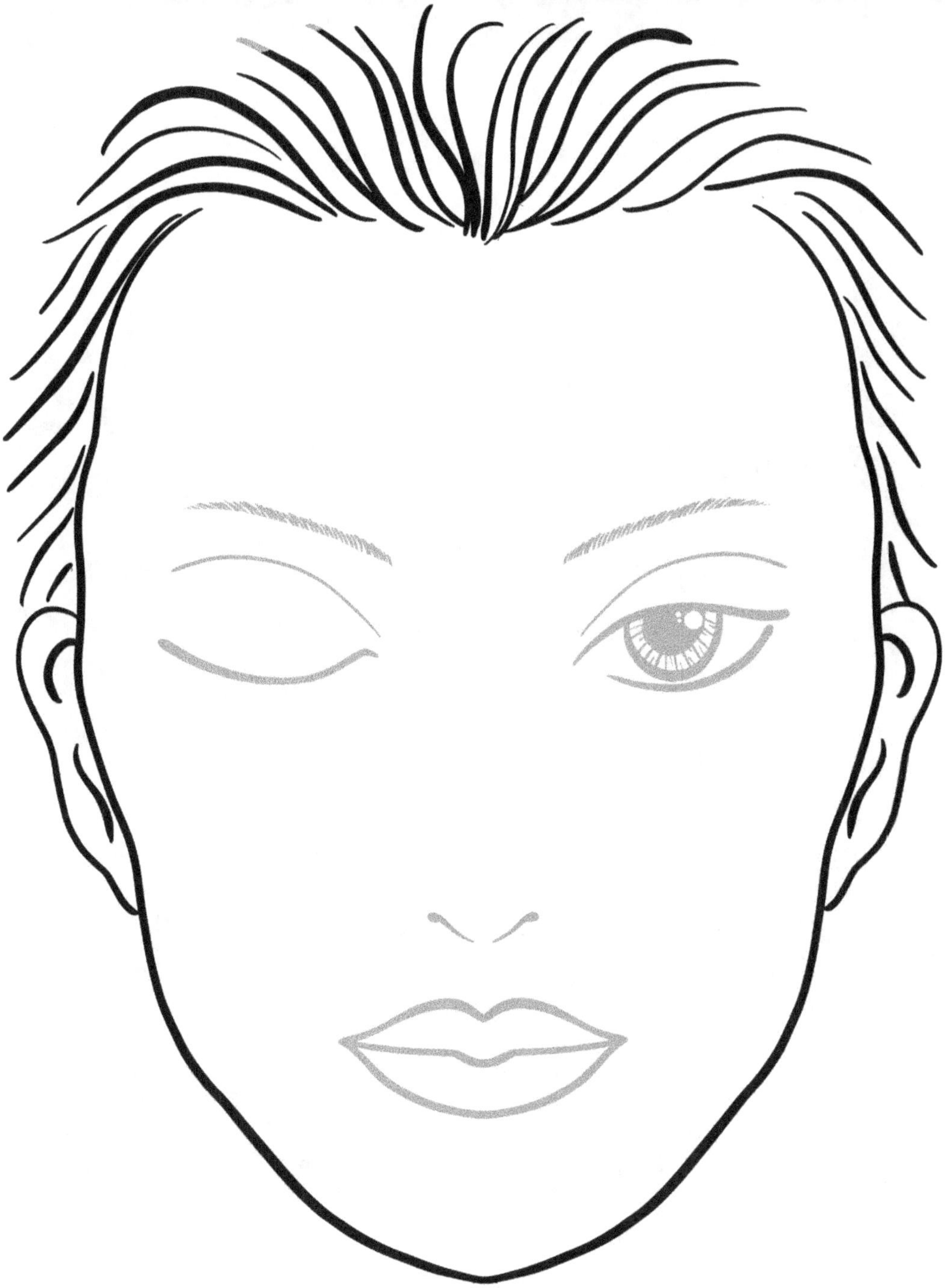

Details

Skin Tone____________________

Eye Color ____________________

Hair Color____________________

Lips (color, brand, etc.)

Lip Liner ____________________

Lip Color ____________________

Gloss ____________________

Eyes (color, brand, etc.)

Brows ____________________

Lid Color 1 ____________________

Lid Color 2 ____________________

Lid Color 3 ____________________

Crease____________________

Eye Liner____________________

Mascara ____________________

Face (color, brand, etc.)

Concealer____________________

Foundation____________________

Contour____________________

Blush ____________________

Highlights ____________________

Powder____________________

Design/Client Name______________ Date______________

Concealer	Foundation	Contour	Blush	Highlights	Powder	Eye Liner	Mascara
Brows	Lid Color 1	Lid Color 2	Lid Color 3	Crease	Lip Liner	Lip Color	Lip Gloss

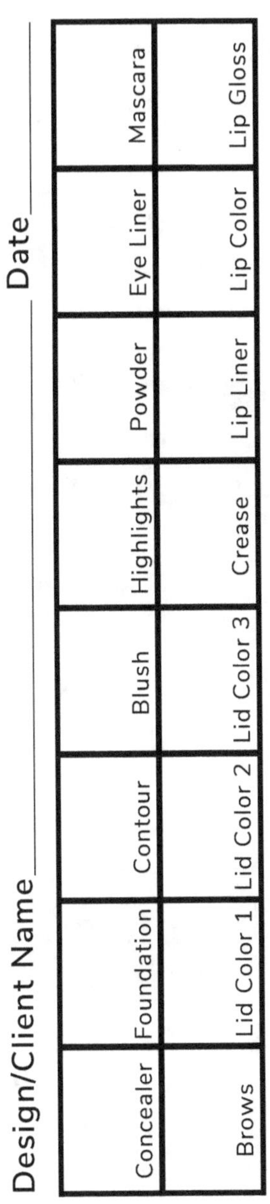

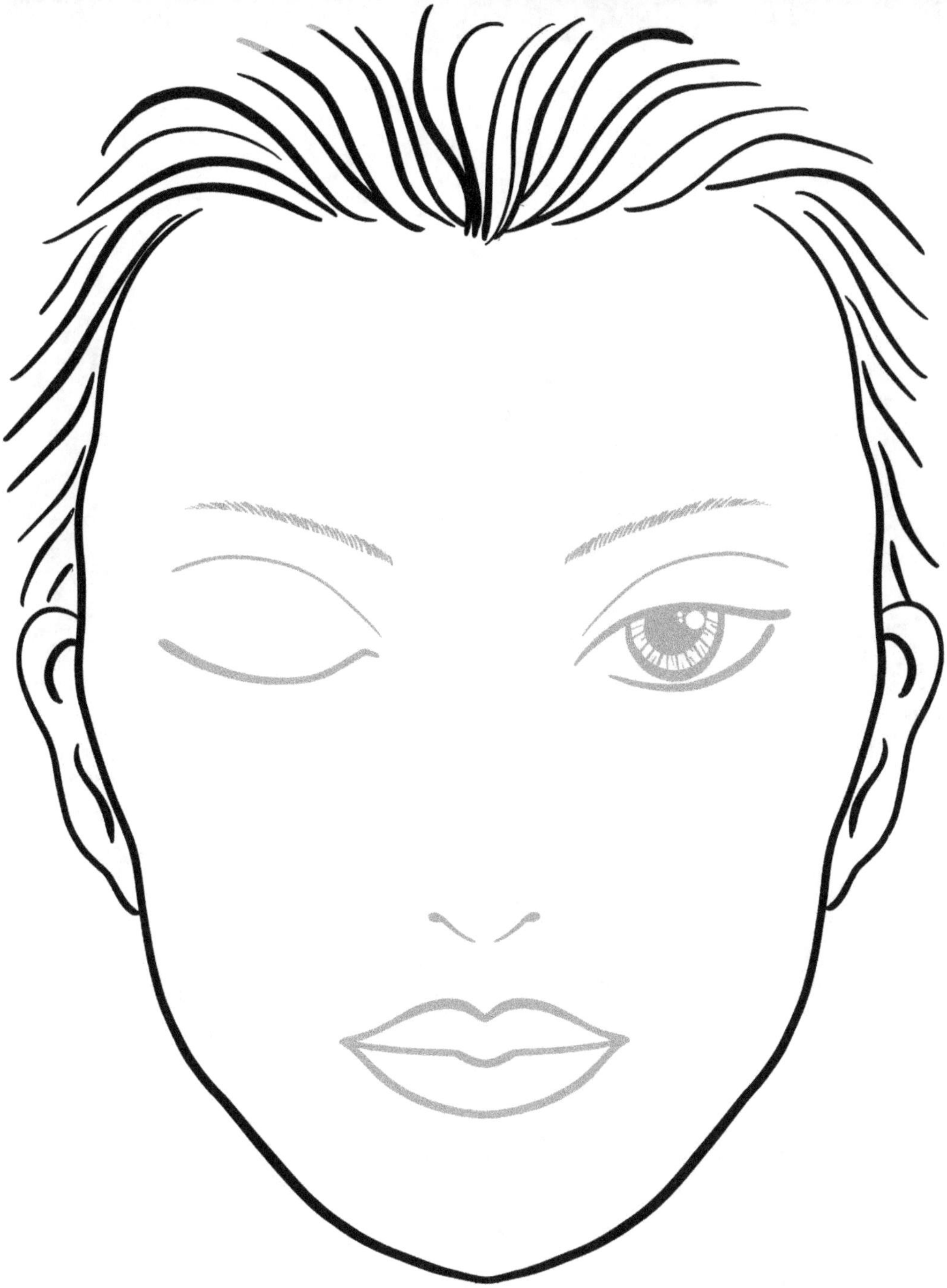

Details

Skin Tone______________________

Eye Color ______________________

Hair Color______________________

Lips (color, brand, etc.)

Lip Liner ______________________

Lip Color ______________________

Gloss ______________________

Eyes (color, brand, etc.)

Brows ______________________

Lid Color 1 ______________________

Lid Color 2 ______________________

Lid Color 3 ______________________

Crease______________________

Eye Liner______________________

Mascara ______________________

Face (color, brand, etc.)

Concealer______________________

Foundation______________________

Contour______________________

Blush ______________________

Highlights ______________________

Powder______________________

Design/Client Name______________ Date______________

Concealer	Foundation	Contour	Blush	Highlights	Powder	Eye Liner	Mascara
Brows	Lid Color 1	Lid Color 2	Lid Color 3	Crease	Lip Liner	Lip Color	Lip Gloss

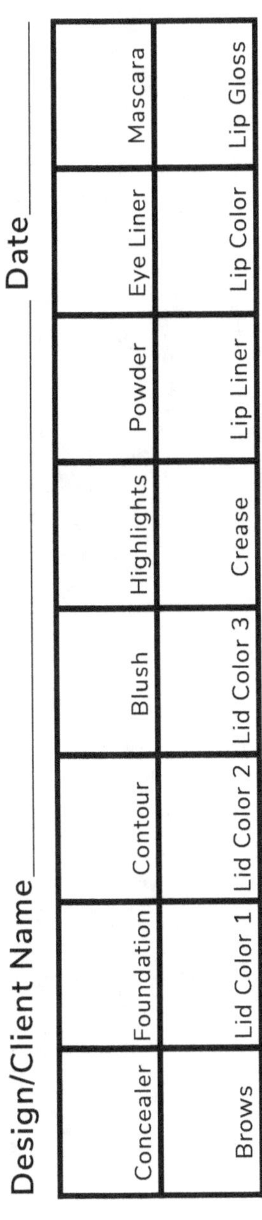

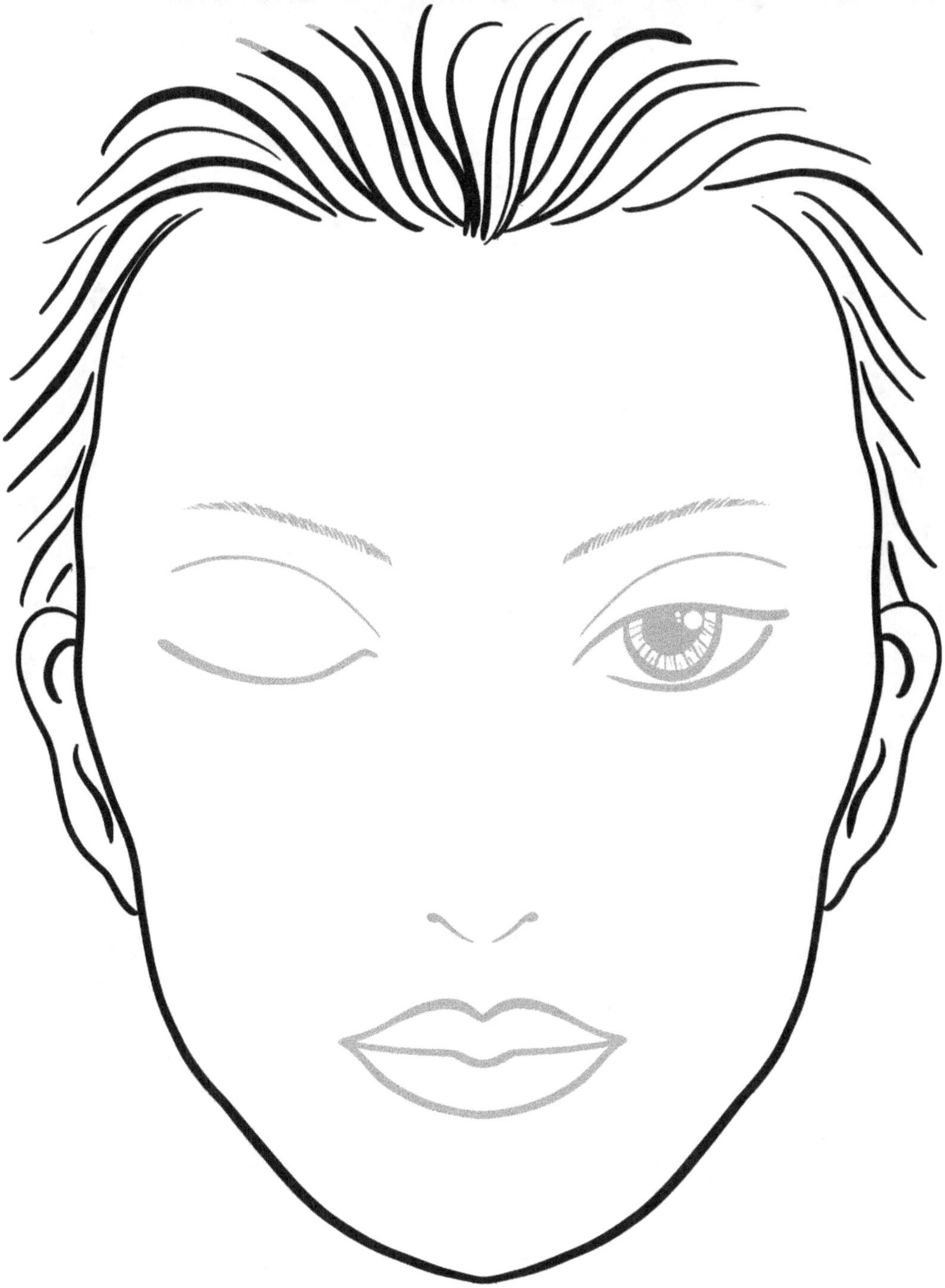

Details

Skin Tone______________________

Eye Color ______________________

Hair Color______________________

Lips (color, brand, etc.)

Lip Liner ______________________

Lip Color ______________________

Gloss ______________________

Eyes (color, brand, etc.)

Brows ______________________

Lid Color 1 ______________________

Lid Color 2 ______________________

Lid Color 3 ______________________

Crease______________________

Eye Liner______________________

Mascara ______________________

Face (color, brand, etc.)

Concealer______________________

Foundation______________________

Contour______________________

Blush ______________________

Highlights ______________________

Powder______________________